HOOKED ON DRAMA

The Theory and Practice of Drama in Early Childhood

SECOND EDITION

KATHLEEN WARREN

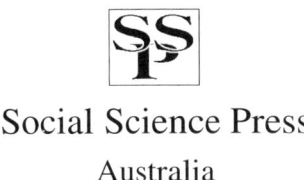

Social Science Press
Australia

Published in 1999 by
SOCIAL SCIENCE PRESS
PO Box 624
Katoomba NSW 2780
(A Division of David Barlow Enterprises Pty. Limited
ACN 001 943 200)
Telephone: (02) 4782-2909 ✻ Fax.: (02) 4782-5303
Email: socsci@ozemail.com.au
Web Site: http://www.ozemail.com.au/~socsci

© Kathleen Warren

ISBN 1 876033 16 9

All rights reserved. This publication is not to be duplicated/or reproduced, either in whole, or in part, in any form whatsoever, without permission from the Publisher.

Should evidence to the contrary arise then the Author and Publisher will pursue their acknowledged rights as stated in Copyright Law.

COVER PHOTOGRAPH BY:
The Photo Library of Australia
Level 1, 7 West Street
North Sydney NSW 2060

Photographer: John Panton

PRINTING BY:
Ligare Pty Ltd
138 Bonds Road
Riverwood NSW 2210

Ritual and ceremony 39

Productive tension 40

CHAPTER FIVE – DIRECTING THE ACTION   43

- *TECHNIQUES AND CONVENTIONS*

  Varying the task 43

  Costumes and props 47

  Scenery 50

  Performing a scene 52

  Dealing with difficult moments 52

  In summary 59

CHAPTER SIX – VARIATIONS ON A THEME   61

- *DIFFERENT STROKES FOR DIFFERENT FOLKS*

  The two-year-olds 61

  Older children 66

  Ethnicity and Multiculturalism 70

  Children with special needs 72

CHAPTER SEVEN – ALARUMS AND EXCURSIONS   81

- *SOME SUGGESTIONS AND A FEW CAUTIONS*

  Popular Culture 81

  The drama space 82

  The size of the group 83

  Going on a journey 84

  Irrelevant asides 84

  Keep the input accurate 85

Contents

PROLOGUE vi

CHAPTER ONE – THE MAGIC OF DRAMA   1

- *INTRODUCTION TO THE ART FORM*
  The foundations of drama in early childhood 2
  What is drama? 3
  What is process drama? 4
  Drama and learning 5

CHAPTER TWO – SETTING THE STAGE   7

- *TOPIC, ROLE AND FOCUS*
  Planning for drama 7

CHAPTER THREE – CURTAIN UP!   21

- *GETTING STARTED*
  How to begin 21
  Past, present and future 23

CHAPTER FOUR – ON WITH THE PLAY   29

- *CO-ORDINATING THE DRAMA*
  Using Language Effectively 29
  Withholding expertise 36
  Delaying into experience 37

Ethics and values 86
Gender equity 87
Reflecting on experience 88

CHAPTER EIGHT – SCRIPT AND TEXT   91

- *SOME LESSON PLANS*
    PLAN ONE 91
    PLAN TWO 98
    PLAN THREE 104
    PLAN FOUR 108
    PLAN FIVE 113
    PLAN SIX 119
    PLAN SEVEN 123

CHAPTER NINE – EPILOGUE   127

- *SOME FINAL THOUGHTS*
    BIBLIOGRAPHY 129

PROLOGUE

My first introduction to what we now refer to as *process drama* came from the film *Three Looms Waiting* which introduced and discussed the work of the British drama educator, Dorothy Heathcote. I was enraptured by the ways in which she and the children with whom she worked, built drama experiences on the ideas, contributions and suggestions of the participants. It seemed to me that the drama episodes woven by Heathcote and her classes were not only theatrically powerful but were developmentally appropriate for children of all ages and abilities, drawing as they did on the fundamental bases of human communication.

I had been involved in theatre as an actor and a director and had taught and adjudicated in the field of Speech and Drama for many years, but was aware that the approach to drama I had followed with students who were interested in performing was inappropriate for my work with young children. Some techniques of improvisation could perhaps be adapted for children in the first years of school but were unsuitable for pre-schoolers and toddlers. The social, emotional, intellectual and theatrical power of Heathcote's work, however, could challenge and engage *all* children.

Since then I have observed and worked with Heathcote, with many of her students and colleagues and with teachers around the world who have been influenced by her. I freely acknowledge the inspiration and encouragement I have had from the work and writings of a multitude of drama practitioners. I recognise too, the assistance I have received from the many early childhood educators who welcomed me into their centres, allowing me to test and develop my ideas with children. It is the children who have been the most important contributors to my work. It is their responses, their ideas to which I constantly refer and it is they who have enabled me to develop my ideas about the theory and practice of drama in early childhood

The first edition of this book was an attempt to share with teachers the ideas and strategies I had found successful and so promote enthusiasm for the art form. Since that time I have continued to work with children and to talk to teachers about their understanding and practice of drama. Many of their suggestions appear in this edition. In particular I would like to acknowledge the contributions of the teachers I interviewed for my doctoral thesis, some of whom I have quoted directly in this book, for the points they made exemplified certain issues so precisely.

This edition echoes and extends the earlier one, presenting a comprehensive account of the forms and contexts of drama pertinent to young children, as well as discussing the modifications needed for diverse ages and stages. The book leads teachers through the strategies involved in planning and implementing successful drama experiences. It begins by recognising drama's foundation in children's sociodramatic play and continues to view the art form as developmentally appropriate practice which has social and educational relevance to young children. Drama is presented as a powerful learning and teaching medium for *all* children regardless of age or ability.

New features in this edition include a discussion of the power of drama for children with special needs, gender equity, ethics and values and drama for a multicultural society. There are additional practical examples and an entirely new set of drama plans together with suggestions as to how these plans can be adapted for a range of ages and abilities. As teachers read this book I hope they will find ideas that will encourage their use of drama.

Through their play, children learn about 'power and responsibility, love and fear' (Haseman and O'Toole, 1986 p.1). They examine social rules, power, control and negotiation (Dau, 1991 p.74; Bolton, 1997), developing strategies which enable them to achieve social competence. Play facilitates problem solving and fosters creativity (Clyde and Fleet, 1993 p.27). As children examine the relationships between real articles and devices and the symbols they choose to represent them (a box for a car, stones for treasure, a scarf for Superman's cloak, a cardboard carton construction for a pirate ship), they develop representational competence. They communicate meaning, particularly non-literal meaning, within the play context as they think and talk about things that are not physically present or in the immediate environment (Perlmutter and Pellegrini, 1989 p.155). As Neelands and Goode (1995 p.42) suggest, playfulness is a term which describes a basic human instinct that involves children (and adults) playing with the relationships between symbols and their normally accepted meanings to create 'new possibilities of meaning'.

Fein's definition of dramatic play, cited in Dau (1991 p.72) emphasises the similarity between play and drama:

> *In pretend play, one object is used as if it were another,*
> *One person behaves as if she were another and an immediate*
> *time and place are treated as if they were otherwise or*
> *elsewhere.*

Sociodramatic play should not be regarded as a developmental stage which engages children as they progress towards 'real' education (Wheeler, 1991 p.11), but as a potent educative force in its own right. Early childhood educators recognise the importance of play in the education of children, but may be less likely to realise that it can lead to planned drama experiences which can extend children's knowledge and understanding. It is children's play experiences which form a firm basis for their willing and able involvement in drama.

WHAT IS DRAMA?

Within the educational context, drama has many forms. The 1998 K-6 Draft Creative Arts Syllabus from the New South Wales Board of Studies provides an encompassing definition.

> *In drama, students enact real and imagined events through the use of*
> *dramatic forms and contexts. Drama provides a means of understanding,*
> *constructing and communicating social, cultural and spiritual values. It*
> *provides for the interpretation and transmission of the past and traditions,*

> *for exploring, celebrating and being challenged by the present and for imagining the future.*
>
> *Drama is a dynamic, collaborative artform that occurs within a framework of contexts:*
>
> - *the 'real' context of personal experiences, cultural backgrounds, environments, attitudes and purposes that participants bring to the drama to explore people, situations, ideas, texts and happenings in the world – the situation of drama.*
> - *the fictional context of the make-believe world that students as participants and audience agree to make together. Within the fictional context, students use role, the elements of drama and the performance elements of theatre. (p. 7)*

Drama begins in babyhood when the baby's carer plays 'Peek-a-boo', or jogs a child up and down while chanting 'Ride-a cock horse'. As children grow, they become involved in making, performing and appreciating drama through a variety of dramatic contexts and forms. Some of the drama forms that can be included in the early childhood curriculum are (in alphabetical order) circus skills, dance drama, dramatic poetry, improvisation (sometimes referred to as creative drama) mask and mime, performance, process drama, puppetry, role play, readers' theatre and story enactment. All can contribute to children's learning and to their enjoyment and understanding of the artform (Warren, 1999 p.3).

This book, however, is particularly concerned with process drama, the 'complex dramatic encounters' (O'Neill, 1995 p.xiii) that are grounded most firmly in children's sociodramatic play, and develop most naturally from it. This is not to say that the other dramatic forms will be ignored, There will be many occasions when they will be a vital part of a process drama experience.

WHAT IS PROCESS DRAMA?

Process drama describes an approach to drama in the classroom that involves children and teacher/s taking roles and through those roles becoming immersed in a fictional situation which occurs and is enacted in the present, in 'now time' as Heathcote puts it. It is concerned with 'making, performing and appreciating' (NSW Board of Studies, 1998) as children and teachers interact and co-operate in partnership, to develop an imaginary context, performing or enacting the evolving, but unpredictable scenario. As children identify with the imagined roles and predicaments, they examine past, present and future experiences, their own and those of others (Norman, 1999 p.9).

As a process drama develops, a story unfolds, although the story is not the important issue. It is what happens as the story evolves that matters. It will, like a good play, be 'well constructed' (Morgan and Saxton, 1987 p.5). There will be an *exposition* where the children and teacher share an understanding of what the drama is to be about, *rising action and complication* where the group examines the problem from different perspectives, the *climax* or crisis where they will come upon the moment or situation which indicates the drama is approaching its peak and finally, the *denouement,* when children have the opportunity to make sense of that significant moment and of the whole experience.

Process drama is not synonymous with theatre, although it incorporates and uses many theatrical techniques. The building of a dramatic world 'an imagined elsewhere with its own characters, locations and concerns' (O'Neill, 1995 p.xi) is a valid description of process drama and of the theatre. The skilful orchestration of the elements of drama, (tension, focus, mood, contrast, symbol, space, sound and silence, stillness and movement, darkness and light) make the artform powerful. Heathcote (1985) points out that in the theatre these elements are used for the effect they have on the audience. In process drama in early childhood they are used to make an impact on the children who are creating the drama.

The ways in which teachers can call on the contexts, elements and forms of theatre and drama to encourage children's engagement in and enjoyment of the artform is the primary focus of this book.

Drama and learning

Dorothy Heathcote, an English drama educator, has been a pioneer in the development of the techniques of drama in the classroom referred to as process drama. Her work, along with that of Gavin Bolton, has had a profound influence on drama education throughout the world. Both Heathcote and Bolton continue to emphasise the ways in which drama can foster children's knowledge and understanding. Heathcote has often been heard to ask teachers about to embark on a drama experience, 'Just what do you want these children to learn?'.

The concept of learning is broad. It is difficult to think of any of life's experiences from which we could not learn something. The learning that can accrue to children through drama is similarly extensive and encompasses cognitive, social, emotional and moral learning, 'the issues of human concern' Carroll,1988 p.58). Any learning that is developmentally appropriate for anyone at any age can be approached through the powerful learning medium of drama. Neelands (1984) has pointed out that it is 'unequivocally child centred'. It draws on children's current knowledge, understanding, interests and language and seeks to extend them.

Drama can foster language development, and can encourage problem solving abilities. It can give children experiences in decision making, and can develop their knowledge and understanding of the past, the present and the future. Drama can increase children's understanding of the complexities of the human condition, and can stretch their imagination. (see Warren, 2000 for a detailed discussion of the ways in which process drama develops children's thinking). It can encourage co-operative behaviour, it can give them experiences in which their opinions and their decisions matter and it can draw on knowledge and understanding which they already have but do not always know they have.

Heathcote (1985) believes that children know and understand things they are barely conscious of knowing or understanding. Drama can act as the catalyst that brings this knowledge and understanding to the surface where it can, at last, be of use to its owners. As Heathcote (1985) says, knowing something is not enough. We must be aware that we know it if it is to be of use to us. Drama enables children to own their own knowledge (Warren, 2000, 127).

Vygotsky (1978) wrote of the zone of proximal development, suggesting that, with help, (Bruner, 1988 p.92 writes of teachers 'scaffolding' the learning) children are able to solve problems and deal with situations which, on the surface, would appear to be beyond them, given their current developmental level. Process drama engages children in fictional situations that lead them towards this zone of proximal development and so to new skills, new knowledge and new understanding.

The following chapters will help teachers develop their own skills in drama. The theory underlying the art form will be integrated with practical suggestions so, as teachers gather ideas about what to do and how to do it they will develop a rationale for the inclusion of drama in the early childhood curriculum.

CHAPTER TWO

SETTING THE STAGE
TOPIC, ROLE AND FOCUS

PLANNING FOR DRAMA

Like all good lessons, process drama is planned. This chapter suggests and discusses four preparatory decisions that need to be made; the topic of the drama, its focus and the roles to be taken by the children and teacher. While the topic of the drama will probably be the first decision made, decisions about roles and focus can be taken in either order. Sometimes the drama's topic leads clearly to its focus, with decisions about roles coming later. On other occasions, the decisions made about the roles for the children and teacher will suggest an appropriate focus.

TOPIC: WHAT WILL THE DRAMA BE ABOUT?

Early childhood educators recognise the importance of developing learning experiences that are appropriate to children's developing interests and abilities. Within these parameters, teachers have many choices when deciding what a drama experience should be about.

Stories and poems

When teachers who are inexperienced in drama think about incorporating it into their teaching, their first thoughts often turn to the stories familiar to the children. This can be an excellent place to begin. Davies (1983, p.23) refers to the school library as a fruitful source of ideas for drama experiences and Booth (1987 p.47) agrees that stories and poems make ideal starting points for drama. Teachers may begin by getting children to act out these stories. However this approach is limited. Children are restricted by the story line, by the characters and in some cases by the dialogue. There is not much scope for original input by either teacher or children.

When children are asked to act out stories, only a few may be involved, with the rest watching. Those who do take roles in the story are likely to be the more confident and out-going children while the shyer, more retiring ones shrink back and hope they will not be asked to take part. These quieter children may well develop the idea that drama is for people who like being centre stage but not something in which they would want to take an active part. Process drama involves all the children at the level at which they chose to be involved, and is an enjoyable and beneficial experience for everyone.

If a process drama is based on a story, the whole story need not be used. The drama can develop from an incident in the story or perhaps a character or characters from the story or even an incident, character or characters who could have been in the story. The story becomes a *pre-text* for the dramatic experience (O'Neill, 1995 p.42). This gives more scope for the development of a drama which has no pre-determined constraints.

Here are a few examples based on stories popular with young children. These examples suggest starting points for drama and also refer to roles which could be taken by the children as well as a role which could be assumed by the teacher. Cooks (children in role) have been hired to provide the banquet for the wedding breakfast for Cinderella and Prince Charming; a messenger from Batman (teacher in role) comes to the police (children in role) because the Batmobile has vanished; Mary, Mary, Quite Contrary (teacher in role) comes to some gardeners (children in role) because her silver bells have turned purple; a troll has taken up residence under a bridge and the farmer (teacher in role) doesn't know what to do; Max's mother (from *The Wild Things* by Maurice Sendak) checks on Max's boat one night and finds a Wild Thing fast asleep. Just about any story can form the basis for a successful drama experience if an episode in the story, or an episode that could have been in the story provides the starting point. Beginning in the middle can be a particularly appropriate and dramatic strategy (O'Neill, 1995 p.137).

Dorothy Heathcote (1984 p.48)) has this to say;

> *Drama is not stories retold in action. Drama is human beings confronted by situations which change them because of what they must face in dealing with those challenges. An open ended situation is easer for teachers who feel themselves to be novices, than a story where the beginning and the end are pre-known.*

Children's interests

Topics for drama can also be developed around some aspect of life in which the children have shown an interest. Early childhood teachers are particularly skilled at observing children and using those observations as the foundations for developmentally appropriate learning. O'Toole (1998 p.8) emphasises the importance of beginning a drama 'where the children are at'. Dunn (1995, p.7) suggests that when a drama is based on something that beguiles children, the work is likely to be 'more passionate, intense and purposeful' simply because the children *are* interested in the topic. Such interests may have arisen through a craze that is sweeping the centre, possibly cultivated by television or other commercial interests. Cartoons, children's entertainers, dinosaurs, heavily advertised toys, superheroes can all provide starting points for effective and engaging drama. A current happening of relevance to the community (bushfires, floods, festivals) can suggest appropriate content. Children's interest in a particular topic or issue may have been fostered by work in which the group has been engaged. Teachers and children may have been discussing farms, under the sea, space travel, holidays, animals, the seasons, festivals, dinosaurs or monsters; such material can be the source of effective drama, provided it has dramatic potential or can have dramatic potential built into it.

Heathcote has been heard to remark that the best dramas are in planets or caves. This does not mean, of course, that these are the preferred settings for drama experiences, but rather that the exotic has more dramatic potential than the mundane. If the topic for the drama is shopping, for example, there is little dramatic potential and little effective learning to be gained by children pushing imaginary trolleys round an imaginary supermarket. However, if the children are cast as support crew for an expedition whose job is to outfit that expedition, then shopping can take on a more extended meaning.

When choosing and developing the topic for a drama, teachers are likely to have specific learning objectives in mind. These can be related to the topic itself. For instance a teacher might want the children to develop knowledge and understanding of a particular subject or issue. A drama about a farm might be used to develop children's knowledge and understanding of why some animals are farmed and not others. If the learning desired is to be on caring for others, the children may need to be framed in a situation in which they have to look after a helpless creature. A lost baby dragon, for example, might need help to find its way home. A drama on dinosaurs could be a vehicle for problem solving. The desired learning might focus primarily on aspects of the art form itself as, through the drama, children are led to recognise the use of role.

The topics of drama and the ways in which those topics can be interpreted will be referred to again and examples will be given as the book proceeds.

Taking roles

Crucial to the concept of process drama is the enactment of a role. In the theatre actors take roles and in process drama so do both children and teachers. It is through these role/s that the children and their teacher 'create and maintain the dramatic worlds' (O'Neill, 1994 p.37).

The role/s for the children

The role/s in which the children are cast depends on the drama itself but a useful rule is to cast the children as people who have the knowledge and expertise to manage the situations that occur as the drama proceeds and who can be called on to suggest effective solutions to problems that arise.

Heathcote (1984, p.205) refers to this technique as Mantle of the Expert where 'the class is set upon a task in such a way that they function as (fictional) experts'. A messenger from Xena, the Warrior Princess (teacher in role) needs builders to work on Xena's castles which are deteriorating (NSW Board of Studies, 1998 p.43). A lady who likes gardening needs expert gardeners who can help her with some problems she is having. Someone who had found a lost baby bird needs ornithologists who can help it; (Warren, 2000), a farmer whose property is being over-run with prickle bushes needs agricultural experts to help solve the problem.

Children do not, of course, have to prove their expertise (Heathcote and Pennington, 1989 p.3; Heathcote and Bolton, 1994 p.173). This would immediately disempower them for they would suddenly become inexpert. Four-year-olds in role as internationally acclaimed chefs who are to prepare the wedding breakfast for Cinderella and Prince Charming could never be expected to take on that task in reality, but drama makes it possible. Empowered by being treated as experts they behave as if they are.

How can young children be regarded as experts and in what? Children can be regarded as experts in anything we choose. By the time children have reached the age of three, they have amassed much knowledge and understanding on which teachers can draw and extend. They can be cast as experts by simply being told that is the role they will take in the drama.

I told some three and four year olds that they would be fire fighters in a drama. Then I entered in role as a new recruit to the fire brigade who wanted to know what being a fire fighter would entail. The detail and complexity of the information they gave me was amazing. On another occasion I cast the children as detectives.

Before I told them the problem (the rainbow had been stolen) I asked them just what sort of work they did as detectives - so I could be sure I had come to the right people. When I did pose the problem of the stolen rainbow, a five year old spoke up. 'Well if the rainbow's gone it means that the sun and the rain have been stolen, because that's what makes the rainbow.'

Just as the topics on which drama can be based are limitless, so are the areas in which children, even very young children, can be designated experts. Here are some of those areas:

- Children are expert in the daily lives of children like themselves. They know what children do and what they are supposed to do.
- They know what constitutes pro and anti-social behaviour in a variety of contexts.
- They have knowledge of the safe things children can do and of the dangerous things they should not do.
- They have knowledge about food.
- They know about the games children play.
- They know about anything they've learnt about in any situation at all, so they can be experts on animals, birthdays, colours, current events, farms, human behaviour, religious and social festivals, the ocean, the seasons, transport, the weather, workers in the community.

Using the technique of mantle of the expert I have cast children as archaeologists, astronauts, builders, chefs, detectives, explorers, gardeners, ornithologists, palaeontologists, police officers, search and rescue workers, zoologists; an endless list.

With young children, it is easier for everyone if they are cast in the same role at the same time. It is better for all the children to be cast as astronauts rather than casting individual children or groups of children in specific subsidiary roles. Young children, particularly those under six, cannot manage group work where different children take on different roles. It causes confusion and the drama becomes fragmented. The children wander around in an aimless way without much idea of what is expected of them and before long they have lost interest and the whole experience disintegrates. (In Chapter Six suggestions are presented for managing some group work with older children).

Sometimes a teacher will choose not to cast the children in any specific role but rather as people to whom the teacher (in role) has come for help of some sort. On other occasions the children's role will be specific. It does tend to give the drama more focus if the children can be cast in precise roles, related to the topic and to the role the teacher will be taking.

The role/s for the teacher

Working in role comes more easily to early childhood teachers than it may do for teachers of older children. Teachers in early childhood work in role without, perhaps, realising it.

Two children are playing hospitals and a teacher says, 'Oh, dear, how sick is your patient? Can you tell me what is wrong, Doctor?' A little girl is 'feeding' her baby. 'Is your baby on to solids now? What do you find she likes to eat?' A group has set up a restaurant and the teacher enters the scene. 'Are you open yet? I'd love a cup of coffee.' Does that sound familiar? Such responses are made by early childhood teachers every day.

Using role in a drama experience differs from spontaneous responses to incidents in children's sociodramatic play. In process drama teachers make deliberate decisions about the role or roles they will take. When teachers take roles in process drama experiences, along with the children, they use a powerful teaching technique which serves to develop and deepen children's understanding of and commitment to the experience and extends the learning that flows from it. It adds to the drama's authenticity, and facilitates a re-negotiation of the normal teacher-child relationship. The teacher can demonstrate what is required in certain situations and can use language that extends children's own use of language (Fleming, 1994 p.99).

When choosing the role for the teacher it is important to consider the relationships of power that are being established. The role chosen should be one which enables the teacher and children to work in partnership. When teachers work in role they are no longer the ones with all the knowledge, in total control, the decision makers but are participants in the fictional context of the drama along with the children. It may appear as if they are in charge, and of course, in a sense they are, for teachers can never relinquish responsibility for the quality of the experience (Heathcote, 1984 p.132). Working in role, however, allows teachers to *guide* the lesson, working at all times to foster the children's construction of meaning.

> *The teacher in role has power but it is not of the conventional kind. It carries within it its opposite; a potential for being powerless....the power relationship between pupils and teacher within the drama is tacitly perceived as negotiable.*
> Bolton (1984) cited in O'Neill (1995 p.62).

The teacher can take a role of high status, of medium status or of low status. The high status role is probably the least useful when working with young children. It might seems as if it has the advantage of controlling the lesson, but this tends to be counter-productive. One of the aims of process drama is to negotiate a transfer of power from the teacher to the children and if the teacher is in a high status role, that is harder to do.

A low status role of someone who needs help is the most effective role the teacher can take when working with young children. During the course of a drama experience the teacher might move in and out of other roles as well and occasionally one or other of these might be of a higher status, although it need not. It all depends on the plan that has been have developed and on the way the drama is progressing, taking into account the contributions of the children.

Consider some roles a teacher might take. One role is that of someone who has just got a new job but doesn't know what will be expected. Some examples of 'new recruit' roles are an astronaut, a caterer, a circus owner, a pirate, an explorer, a farmer, a fire-fighter, a gardener, a pirate, a queen. The teacher can be someone related to a story or rhyme; Little Bo Peep, the giant's wife (from Jack and the Beanstalk), Goldilock's mother, Mr Gumpy. Another useful role is that of messenger or go-between (Morgan and Saxton, 1987 p.42). I have found this a most effective role in dramas about the super-heroes. A messenger from Superman cannot be expected to have Superman's skills and knowledge but is able to relay messages. Alternatively the teacher can be what Morgan and Saxton (p.43) have referred to as 'one of the gang', someone who has no special role or status but who is working alongside the children to solve whatever problem they are facing. Contradictory roles can also be effective. Davies (1983 p.41) recommends 'the apparently incongruous or paradoxical' (the reluctant dragon, the unhappy king, the timid pirate, the gardener whose plants always die, the mountain climber who is afraid of heights) as having immediate dramatic potential.

The important issue is the relationship between the role the children take and the role the teacher adopts. The drama is most likely to achieve success if the children are cast in the roles of the ones with the expertise and the teacher as the one who needs their advice and assistance.

This raises the issue of bonding. It is important that the children develop a bond with the character who asks for their assistance so they feel they *want* to help. If no bonding takes place, the children feel no commitment to the character and are not particularly interested in helping solve his or her problems. When bonding occurs, the rest of the drama is much more likely to fall into place (Heathcote, 1985). Bonding is more inclined to develop if the children believe that their actions, suggestions and decisions matter.

Using other adults in role

When teachers work with young children it is often useful to plan to cast another adult (or adults) in role as the drama progresses. The role/s of the other adult/s depends on the situation but two types of role may be particularly useful. The teacher could cast the second adult as someone who has already been referred to. I took the role of a castle owner who had hired a monster (another adult in role) to guard my castle while I was away. Unfortunately this monster was extremely timid and hid whenever the castle was threatened. By casting another adult as the timid monster, the group could travel with me to the castle and see the timid monster for themselves. The advantage of this is that the children are not trying to solve the problem through the owner of the castle but can work directly with the monster. A plan for this lesson appears in the K-6 Creative Arts Draft Syllabus Support Document (NSW Board of Studies, 1998 p.15).

Another adult can enter the drama in the role designated by Morgan and Saxton (1987 p.45) as one who is opposed to the group. One of my students developed a drama experience in which the children had to climb a mountain to get a special plant that could be used to cure disease. The teacher had put the children in role as mountain climbers and herself as someone who wanted a plant that grew on the mountain because this plant would cure her mother's sickness.

She asked the mountain climbers about their experiences in mountain climbing, so she would know she had come to the right people, and when she was satisfied as to their expertise, they all set off. On reaching the top of the mountain, they were confronted by another adult in role as someone who lived on the mountain and who had no intention of allowing them to pick any special plants that grew there. The children then had the problem of deciding how best to deal with this person who was determined to thwart their plans.

It is possible for the teacher to change roles and to become the person opposed to the group and if no other adults are available this might be the only way of introducing such a character. This will not confuse young children provided it is clearly signalled. After all, it is what children do in their own dramatic play 'I will drive the truck and you will help me unload the parcels. Now I will be a police officer and you can drive the truck and I will tell you where to park it.' 'I am skiing at the dam and I fall in and you have to rescue me. Now you can drive the ambulance and I will be the doctor and she can be the person who is hurt.'

In a drama experience it is important that the children realise that these changes in role are about to take place. The teacher might say, 'Now I'm going to be someone else in our drama. I'll just go over here and when I come back, I won't be the lady whose mother is sick. I'll be somebody else'. Walking a few steps away from the children and returning immediately, the teacher signals by what he or she says just what the new role is. 'What are you mountain climbers doing on my mountain? This is my mountain and everything on it belongs to me.'

I watched Cecily O'Neill (O'Neill,1990) take the role of a pathetic ogre's wife who had eaten only bread and cheese since her husband chased Jack down the beanstalk and was killed when Jack cut it down. Then, just as the children would have felt sorry for her and inclined to help, she let it be known that she did have a child in a cage out the back and was saving it for her birthday tea. The children could be asked to decide on the gender, name and age of this child.

The question could be asked, either by the character or by a teacher facilitator, taking the role Morgan and Saxton (1987 p.45) have called 'devil's advocate', 'Well, would it really matter if she ate this one child? It seems awful that she hasn't got anything nice for her birthday.' The teacher would hope that the children (or at least one of them) would refute the suggestion and would explain that eating people is not allowed.

There is a danger that the children will agree. If this happens there are several courses of action open to the teacher. Going along with them and agreeing that the ogre's wife could eat the child would not sit happily with most teachers. I know it would not sit happily with me. The teacher might go into role as the child who is about to be eaten and plead the case. The teacher could go out and re-enter in role as the child's mother who is appalled at the idea that her child should be eaten. She can talk about how much she loves the child and how much she wants it back! If there is a spare adult (or two) available they can take one or both of these roles. If the teacher does not want to introduce other characters at this point he or she could say (as if still mulling over the problem), 'On the other hand, I suppose a mother might be sad if her child was eaten. Who would tell her, do you think?'

When another adult is in role, or if the teacher takes a new role, it can be helpful if the children are asked to direct that adult in gesture, movement and perhaps dialogue suited to the role. In a drama about a dinosaur who had lost her egg, I told the children that their teacher would be taking the role of a dinosaur and asked which sort of dinosaur they would suggest. Accepting the suggestion with most support (usually a pterodactyl) I asked the children to show the teacher how to stand and move in that role and the teacher followed their directions. This empowers the children for they are creating and so controlling what could be a frightening character. It can also be helpful for the character to move in out of the role a few times. 'Can you show us what you are like when you are a pterodactyl?' Let the adult assume the role for a few seconds. 'Now show us what you are like when you are Pat.' At this point, Pat behaves as normal. 'Now show us what you are like when you are the pterodactyl' and so on back and forth three or four times. A plan for this lesson can be found in the K-6 Draft Creative Arts Syllabus Support Document (NSW Board of Studies, 1998 p.23).

The bridge between fantasy and reality can be fragile for young children and they may need help in building belief in the fictional context. It is not unusual for a child to say, 'That's not really a pterodactyl – it's really Pat.' The answer here is, 'Yes, usually that person is Pat, but today in our drama Pat is being a pterodactyl', and be prepared to repeat this as many times as necessary.

In process drama the children are participants in the ongoing action. There is an 'immediacy and spontaneity' (O'Neill, 1995 p.90) which encourages their belief and participation in the experience. The role/s in which they are cast and the role/s taken by the teacher are critical.

Some thoughts about role

When casting the children, teachers should be careful to avoid gender specific terminology. Use the term police officers rather than police men and women, fire fighters, not firemen. Luckily, most role titles can apply to both men and women. In the main, teachers should take roles appropriate to their gender. It is inconsistent for a man to take the role of Mary who lost her lamb, but he could play her brother or father. As a woman, I would take the role of an Empress rather than an Emperor. When women adopt male roles it can emphasise the idea that only men can take exciting or important roles. It is usually possible to find a suitable female role that is compatible with the drama's intent.

The significance of letting children know what is happening when an adult is changing role has already been mentioned. However, there will be times when the teacher needs to step out of the role for organisational purposes. Perhaps there is a need to introduce or explain some aspect of the drama. The children may have suggested the need for a cave. The teacher, coming out of role, might ask for suggestions. 'What could we use for a cave do you think?' If a table is suggested, there may be a need for the teacher and children to set the scene. It is not necessary for the teacher to explain he or she is reverting to being the teacher or facilitator. The children are well able to understand and accept this change in demeanour and speech. Once the task has been completed, the teacher resumes the role and the drama continues. If matters of discipline arise, these too can be dealt with out of role.

When another adult takes a role in the drama it can, at times, be particularly powerful if that character does not speak. In a drama where the teacher (working as facilitator) introduced a lost bird, the bird communicated only through mime, gesture and facial expression. The children are impelled to pay close attention to the character so they can understand what it is trying to tell them.

Occasionally an adult in role will overact. This is better avoided than dealt with after it happens for the effects on the drama tend to be disastrous. When an adult takes a role for the first time it is advisable for the teacher to be very clear about what is required of that person. Usually, the adult in role should play the part quietly, taking the lead from the teacher/facilitator. The adult's role is to serve the needs of the drama and of the children, not to display their skills as an actor or to have a bit of fun.

A teacher describes what happened when an adult in role did not understand what was required of her. The children were in role as astronomers who had found a lost star and who had decided it would be returned to the sky. Another teacher was in role as the lost star.

> *She was not really aware of her role. I did explain to her briefly that she would be lost. She would be lying down on the ground and we would find her and we'd think of various modes to get her back in the sky and see what happened. But the teacher went flying off into a cupboard and the children went beserk...she ran into a storage cupboard and twenty children followed her!*
>
> (Ashton, 1996).

Faced with a situation in which the inappropriate acting of an adult in role seems set to destroy the drama, all the teacher can do is try to retrieve the situation. A narrative section might help, moving along to another scene in which the adult does not appear. 'The astronauts sat down and wondered what they had done to frighten the star.' The teacher/facilitator could then instruct the star to come out of role for a while and continue, 'Perhaps we can talk about how we can help her so she knows we do not want to chase her away.' Perhaps the scene can be replayed with the teacher instructing the adult as to what is wanted. 'Well, that was exciting, wasn't it,' the teacher says (through clenched teeth), 'I wonder if we could do that bit again. Sit very quietly, Star and listen to the astronaut's ideas. Perhaps if we watch you carefully, you could smile if you like the idea and look worried if you don't think it is going to work.'

When such misunderstandings occur it is usually because the adult does not realise what is expected. It is better not to use an adult who seems incapable of taking a role effectively.

There are roles for the children and roles that are more appropriately taken by an adult. When an adult takes a role in process drama, the job of that adult is to meet the needs of the children. It is necessary to listen carefully to what the children are saying and interact with them so as to forward the course of the drama. Children cannot do this and it is unfair of the teacher to ask it of them. Small children have difficulty in meeting their own needs; they cannot take on the needs of the rest of the class.

If a teacher does put a child in role, it is likely that he or she will go off on an agenda which will have nothing to do with where the drama is heading. It might be possible to use older children in role on occasion if they understand exactly what is required of them. For instance, if working with five-year-olds, the teacher might be able to use a twelve-year-old in a role in the drama. However, it is unrealistic to expect children of any age will be able to extend younger children or to meet their needs as adults should be able to do.

Focus

Focus refers to the way in which the idea or topic is translated into dramatic action (O'Neill, 1995 p.43) and is related both to the learning potential of the experience and the actual development of the drama. The teacher needs to consider just how the lesson will develop to meet the learning objectives while involving the children in the dramatic encounter. A problem or problems central to the drama need to be considered. A drama lacking focus is unlikely to progress for the experience is likely to be bland and lacking challenge. The drama needs to work toward an issue (or issues) which the children will confront.

Christmas was approaching and a teacher decided to involve her group of two-and-a half to three year olds in a drama that would draw on their interest in the festival. Santa Claus had sent the group a letter to say he had taken Mrs Claus to Fiji on holidays for Christmas and had no-one to deliver the presents. The letter asked the group if they knew of anyone who could help. The children agreed that they and their teacher could be Santa's helpers. The focus of the drama, then, centred on the need to deliver all the presents in just one night.

A group of four-year-olds had been studying the topic of farms and the teacher wanted to involve them in a drama that would draw on and extend their knowledge and understanding of the subject. Cast as agricultural advisers, their task was to advise and assist a dairy farmer (teacher in role) whose paddocks were overgrown with prickle bushes, thus destroying the food supply for her dairy herd. The focus of this drama involved the agricultural advisers in solving the problem of the damaged pastures.

A class of six-year-olds had been investigating the topic of needs and wants. The drama's focus was on the rescue of a baby dragon (teacher in role) who had somehow got lost and on the ways she would have to be cared for until she could be safely reunited with her family (Warren, 2000 p.131).

Additional examples should further clarify the ideas of topic, role/s and focus presented in this chapter as essential initial decisions when planning a drama experience.

A teacher decided to engage her group in a drama experience that would encourage their belief in a fictional context and would engage them in innovative and imaginative thought. She decided that the drama would be about a lost star. The children (as themselves) came upon a lost star (teacher in role). The focus of the drama was for the group to decide how the star could be returned to its rightful place.

Some pre-schoolers had been learning about snakes and lizards. The teacher decided on a drama that would draw on and extend the children's knowledge and understanding of the topic. She put them in role as herpetologists and herself in role as a zoo-keeper who wanted to extend her reptile collection. The focus of the drama engaged the group in accompanying the zoo-keeper on an expedition to a place where snakes and lizards could be found.

Another teacher had observed a high level of verbal aggression in her centre. While there was no physical aggression, there was evidence of emotional hurt as a result of the aggression. She decided that this would be the topic of a drama. The group met a child (teacher in role) who was very upset because one of the Power Rangers had been calling her names and hurting her feelings. The teacher decided that the focus of the drama would engage the group in solving this dilemma. The children decided they would visit the Power Ranger (another adult in role), confront this person with the consequences of the verbal aggression and demand a change of conduct, demonstrating acceptable social behaviour.

Having chosen the topic for the drama experience, the focus or problem and the roles the adults will assume as well as the roles the children will take, the teacher is now ready to consider some of the techniques which will help the lesson succeed.

CHAPTER THREE

CURTAIN UP!

GETTING STARTED

How to begin

When beginning a drama lesson it is important that the children know they are embarking on a fictional journey. Heathcote and Bolton (1994 p.25) emphasise that the word *if* or the implication of if should be introduced early. Chapter Two introduced the fragility of the bridge between fantasy and reality and the younger children are, the more fragile it is so it is wise to begin by making it clear that in drama both the teacher and the children are working in an imaginary context.

I find that a straightforward approach is best. With the children sitting in a circle or in a gathered group, whichever is familiar to them, the teacher can sit with them and say, 'Today we are going to do some drama and when we do drama we can be people who are different from the people we usually are and we can go to different places without ever leaving this room.' It is possible to extend this statement by saying, 'So today in our drama you won't be the children at this kindergarten but you'll be people in the drama. I won't be myself, either and neither will Sandy (naming another adult who will be taking a role/s in the drama). We'll be people in the drama, too.' This may be a useful opportunity to tell the group of the role they will take in the drama. 'And in our drama today you are going to be ornithologists, people who know a lot about birds.' It is advisable to get the children's agreement on this point. 'Is that all right? Would you agree that in our drama today you will be ornithologists, people who know a lot about birds?'

Two points emerge here. One refers to the use of the correct vocabulary when casting children in professional roles. As the example indicates, a term that may be new to children can be covered by slipping in a definition. The use of the correct word, which should be used throughout the drama, adds to the children's knowledge of language. It also serves to add status to the role.

The second point stresses the importance of getting the children's agreement that they will accept the role that has been suggested. Children almost always agree. In the unlikely event that they suggest a different role it may well be one that can be incorporated into the drama planned. If it is not, the teacher must make that clear. I would say, 'Birds. I suppose you could. The trouble is that in our drama today you will need to be people who can talk and who can help me with a problem I have and birds can't do that. So in the drama today, will you all agree to be ornithologists, people who know about birds?'

I am not sure after these initial explanations just how clear young children will be as to the nature of drama. Perhaps it does not matter. The teacher has set the ground rules and it is easy to refer back to them when it becomes necessary. Children's unfamiliarity with the word 'drama' is not a reason for the teacher not to use it, either. We learn new words by hearing others use them in context. Referring to what is being done as drama means the children will immediately discover one definition of the word and that is a good start. If teachers confine their vocabulary to the words they know children understand, they are likely to have rather limited vocabularies and the children with whom they are working will be denied opportunities to extend their own understanding of language.

When working with children in the early school years I might begin the drama lesson by asking them for their understanding of the artform. Typical responses are as follows: 'You do a play', 'It's acting', 'It's like on TV' 'You do mime'. All suggestions can be accepted and can be summarised by the definition already discussed.

Some teachers use the word 'pretending' when they introduce a drama experience. I do not, because, once teachers and children begin a drama, it becomes more than 'pretending', it becomes a genuine and involving experience, so, to me, 'pretending' is not a true description of what will happen. Being a pirate in a drama is not the same as pretending to be a pirate. If the teacher asks the children to assume a role and lets them know that he or she will also be in role, there is a deeper level of involvement than if children are asked to pretend to be that person. Imagining is usually a better word than pretending. Of course, if a child introduces the word by saying, 'We're pretending, aren't we!' then it is best to agree. It is a matter of being open with the children about the fictional nature of the enterprise.

Heathcote and Bolton (1994 p.27) regard such teacher talk as 'raising the curtain, inviting the class to take a peep at the metaphorical stage'. Most young children are well able to understand and accept this invitation. What they are being offered is, as we have already seen, similar to their own experiences in sociodramatic play. Sometimes, however, the reality/fantasy divide is too difficult and the teacher must step in to reassure children.

In a drama in which the children had been cast as travel consultants (the topic was 'holidays') the teacher had taken the role of a customer who wanted advice about an exciting holiday. The group made several suggestions, and one boy suggested 'Africa'. Recognising that such an exotic location offered promising dramatic possibilities, the teacher (still in role as the customer) expressed interest but asked if the travel consultants would come with her. There was general agreement. The teacher noticed, however, that one small girl was aghast! Her lip was trembling and it was obvious that she had not understood that the group would be working in a fictional context. The teacher realised that this difficulty must be dealt with immediately.

Coming out of role, she spoke directly to the child and used the word 'pretending'. 'You know, we are not really going to Africa. We will just pretend to go. We won't really leave this room. Do you think you would like to pretend along with the rest of us?' The child shook her head. 'That's all right', said the teacher. 'You can watch us and when you want to be a part of what we are doing, just join in.' Eventually, after watching the drama progress for some time, the girl rejoined the group. Children cannot be forced to believe in an imaginary context and must be allowed to take their own time to accept a fictional situation.

PAST, PRESENT AND FUTURE

A drama experience begins by letting the children know what has happened in the past to lay the foundations for the present state of affairs. What happens in the drama will lead to a future result, Process drama is always set in the here and now. Even if the teacher is working around an historical incident or has used as a starting point a story set in the past, the drama always happens in what Heathcote calls *now time*. As a drama begins, children are invited to further examine the present and to construct the future, all working together to determine the outcome.

Consider just how the action can begin. The first examples assume that the children are verbal and for most children, verbal fluency is established by the age of three. Chapter Six will consider strategies that can be used with children whose verbal skills are still developing.

The teacher leaves the scene, returning in role after telling the group that this is what will occur. 'I'm just going over there and when I come back, I won't be myself. I'll be someone in the drama.' On return the character explains the situation to the group, usually communicating his/her own role in the process. In a drama about a castle owner who had hired a monster to guard the castle, the teacher in role clarifies that the people he/she meets are psychologists, people who know a lot about why some people are frightened. This is an alternate role for the children to the one suggested in the plan outlined in the K-6 Creative Arts Draft Syllabus Support document (NSW Board of Studies, 1998 p.15). The teacher 'sees' the group and says, 'Excuse me, I'm looking for the psychologists, people who know a lot about why people are frightened.'

Usually, the group will agree that they are those people, providing, of course, that this introduction to their role has taken place earlier. If the teacher is met with blank faces, it is helpful to refer to the earlier discussion. 'Do you remember how we said that when you do drama you can be people who are different to the people you usually are?' The children are likely to agree. 'And do you remember that in the drama today we agreed that you will be psychologists, people who know a lot about why some people are frightened?' Again, the children are likely to agree albeit tentatively. 'Well, I'll just go over here again and when I come back, I won't be myself. I'll be looking for the psychologists and that will be you, won't it?'

It is important to ensure that, at this stage, the children have sufficient understanding of what is happening to enable the drama to proceed. It is worth taking time to establish the children's acceptance of their role/s. Repeating the procedure achieves that. There are rarely any problems the second time around.

The next step is an important one. It involves getting the children to define their terms. If they are in role as people who understand why others are timid, it is necessary for the teacher to listen to their ideas. If, later in the drama, another adult takes the role of the timid monster, these earlier contributions from the children will enable this adult to build the character and dialogue, reflecting the children's previous statements. This is empowering and affirming for children. If a child has said, during the preliminary discussion, that people are frightened of loud noises, the monster can mention this as one of the reasons it is so timid. The owner of the castle can turn to the child who made the suggestion and say 'That's just what you said!'

If the children's knowledge seems scrappy it does not matter. If they can only suggest one or two reasons for people being frightened, the teacher need not worry and more importantly, should not take the opportunity to add to their knowledge by asking questions like, 'Well what about the dark? Some people are frightened of the dark.' Accept whatever the children give. I can promise that, as the drama proceeds, the children's store of knowledge will be activated and more information will come from them.

Now is the time to introduce the teacher's own role (if it has not happened before this) and to introduce the problem or focus of the drama. Using the drama about a timid monster as an example, the teacher might say, 'I'm glad I found you because you do seem to know quite a lot about why people are frightened. Let me tell you my problem. I bought a castle for myself, but I don't get there very often so they said I should find a monster who would live there and scare away intruders. So I did, but it is of no help at all. It is just so timid and frightened. The castle has been robbed twice, because whenever anyone come near, that monster hides and I just don't know what to do.'

The teacher should pause here and listen to and accept any comments the group make. Still in role the teacher can continue, 'So they said, I should find some psychologists because they might be able to help me.' Who are *they*? Well, no-one really, but the phrase is a useful one. It refers to some vague authority whose advice is being heeded. Similar phrases are 'they do say' and 'I have heard' which can be used to introduce information and ideas into the drama without it appearing to have come directly from the teacher. (Heathcote, 1985).

At this point in the lesson, the teacher has explained the past and introduced the present. The past can also be described by a letter that is delivered, just as the teacher is explaining what drama is about. An example was given earlier about a letter sent by Santa Claus, seeking assistance. The information can also be relayed by audio tape. The advantage of a tape, as far as young children are concerned, is that they can listen to what is said, although they may not be able to read a letter which has to be read to them. In a drama about underwater pollution, a tape arrived from a mermaid (complete with watery sound effects) asking for assistance. When using a tape it is a good idea to record the message three times. This avoids the problems of having to rewind and replay the message. The actual delivery of the letter or tape can build excitement and tension, particularly if the teacher/ facilitator regards it, initially, as an unwelcome interruption.

Sometimes it is interesting to begin a drama with an adult in role already in place. The teacher can still indicate that this person will be playing a role in the drama. 'We'll just go over there and when we come back, Chris will be someone special in our drama.' If costume or props are involved the character can don them with the help of the group. This is particularly important for very young children or for children who are developmentally delayed. To confront some children with a character in costume can be terrifying. If, on the other hand, the children have helped transform the character, they have helped create a new identity and are more able to accept it as the drama proceeds.

The group can be taken to the other side of the room while the character settles into position. When the group returns, the drama commences. The teacher might decide to have the character asleep. This can be a useful beginning to a drama experience for young children as it enables them to accept the new character in their own time, As the group returns to the scene, all eyes will be on this 'new' person. The teacher, participating in the drama as teacher/facilitator need not have a defined role. Questions such as 'I wonder who this can be?' 'What is it doing?' 'I wonder why it is here?' can be asked. Someone is likely to observe it is asleep. 'Is it? What do you think we should do?' While all this is going on, the teacher needs to protect the person in role by keeping the children at a reasonable distance. 'It's better not to get too close to strangers.' Eventually someone is sure to suggest waking the character. The teacher can say, doubtfully, 'Wake it up? How would we do that, do you think?'

As suggestions are offered they can be tried out. Children are likely to begin by suggesting some physical contact; tap it, tickle it, stroke it. Get the child who made the suggestion to try. 'Well, you go and tap it and see what happens.' Do not allow all the children to descend en masse. It is the teacher's job to protect an adult in role, especially one who is vulnerable. The teacher continues to take the children's suggestions and provide the means for them to be tried out. If the suggestion is something that everyone can do together (like calling our 'Wake up!') well and good. If it is not, the child who made the suggestions can try it out, but not too roughly. The teacher should not agree to suggestions that are dangerous but need not reprove the child who proposes it. I once had a fairy asleep on the floor and we were considering ways to wake her up. One little boy said, 'We could pick her up and drop her.' I expressed concern. 'But that might hurt her and I don't want to do that.' A popular Australian group of children's entertainers 'The Wiggles' sometimes ask their pre-school audience for advice when one of their number falls asleep on stage. If violent suggestions are made, they never admonish the child who has made that suggestion, but simply point out that they don't want to hurt the character.

Introducing an adult in role in this way provides a slow beginning during which tension builds. The character should not wake too quickly, so the teacher/facilitator needs to arrange with the adult beforehand that there will be a clear verbal signal when this is to happen. The teacher needs to 'read' the children to judge when it is the right moment for the character to wake and signal accordingly. 'I think this will work. I have a feeling that this will work', then the character can 'wake' slowly and look around.

Alternatives to the character being asleep is to have that person looking for something, or just sitting still, looking sad or crying softly provided this is not overdone. When the children have managed to get the character's attention he or she is able to present the situation and begin the action. If one of these introductions to the drama are used, the teacher can take the role although it would not be wise for a lone teacher to begin the drama asleep.

Costumes, objects or pictures can prove useful stimuli that will get a drama started. I once observed a teacher who began by showing the children a picture of a hot-air balloon. She asked, 'I wonder what it would feel like to go on a journey in a hot air balloon' 'I wonder where you could go?' 'I wonder what you'd find when you got there?' Having captured the children's interest and having encouraged them to consider, predict, explain and hypothesise, she was then able to say, 'In our drama today, we could go for a ride in one.'

The teacher might show the children an object. 'I wonder who would wear a necklace like this?' 'I wonder who would drink out of this cup?' Davies (1983) emphasises the importance of using questions to lead into the drama, questions that will challenge children's thought and imagination.

It is the opening scene that provides the momentum for the work. If the topic is presented effectively, the children will be enticed into the drama and will approach the experience with enthusiasm. The children are invited to take an active part in an exciting venture in which their ideas and suggestions will be of utmost importance.

CHAPTER FOUR

ON WITH THE PLAY

CO-ORDINATING THE DRAMA

It might appear that devising and implementing a drama experience is a complicated balancing act. The drama does need to be carefully planned or there is a risk of losing direction with resultant chaos when it comes to the lesson. On the other hand, the plan should be sufficiently open to allow for the children's ideas that will determine and influence the course of the drama. These contributions to the flow of the drama are essential to its success for children will have no commitment to a drama that has no room for their ideas and the course of which seems to have been pre-determined by the teacher. Heathcote emphasises, nevertheless, that a teacher can never get away with shabby planning. Planning provides (Morgan and Saxton, 1987 p.169) 'the invisible safety net when you appear to be working without one.'

As teachers make decisions about topic, role and focus, determining how the lesson will be introduced, they also plan how to engage children in the ongoing experience. What decisions can the children be asked to make? What problems can be posed? How can the teacher make use of the children's ideas to forward the course of the drama? The language of the drama classroom together with the pedagogic skill of questioning will support teachers here.

USING LANGUAGE EFFECTIVELY

Wagner (1976) refers to the various language registers available to teachers and suggests that the register chosen can serve to empower or disempower children. The language interactions between adults and children that take place in drama should cultivate a discussion between equals, in which the children's ideas and opinions are sought and accepted. Heathcote's advice (cited in Carroll, 1988 p.19) is perceptive.

> *In drama you can't talk to the participants with a status attitude like teachers talk to children. You've got to use a language code of choice, and an amount of elaboration in the language that makes them feel like they know what they are doing.*

QUESTIONING

Process drama encourages teachers to use the discourse of questioning (referred to by Morgan and Saxton (1991 p.ix) as 'an essential democratic skill') to empower children and not, as often happens in schools, to disempower them. Bruner (1990 p.26) discusses the value of 'pragmatic, perspectival questions' in enabling people to understand their culture. The examples he suggests ('What would it be like to believe that?' or 'What would I be committing myself to if I believed that?') are exactly the sorts of questions that are asked in process drama, questions which enable children to clarify their thinking (Makin, et al, 1995 p.29). When teachers question as if they really want to know, children are immediately empowered as they recognise they are free to contribute a range of ideas and possible solutions without fear of disapproval or rejection (Warren, 2000 p.130).

Disempowering questions are likely to be asked in such a way as to suggest to children that there is a correct or required answer. Children are disempowered by this approach for, if they are unsure of what the teacher wants by way of response, they are immediately placed in a defensive position. Posing questions as if they appear to be a genuine search for information or ideas is less threatening to children. A tone of voice and choice of language that *invite* children to respond are better options than language that *expects* them to do so, or is so interpreted by the children.

Most teachers are familiar with open and closed questions and may have been taught that open questions are good and closed questions are not productive. Closed questions have only 'yes' or 'no' answers or answers that are tightly proscribed. Open questions allow children to respond more fully. Both open and closed questions have their place in a drama experience but drama also demands questions to which the answer is unknown until the children provide it. A closed question might ask, 'What did the bears have for breakfast?' while an open question might challenge the children's thinking further. 'I wonder why Goldilocks thought it was all right to go into the bear's house?'

Process drama enables questions to be posed to which there are no right or wrong answers, questions which free children to imagine, to reflect, to predict, to hypothesise, to reason, to theorise and to evaluate (Schaffner, 1984). Tough (1977) found that children who are at risk educationally are those who are less efficient in using language for such purposes. She explains that competence in language use is essential for the development of cognitive skills, social awareness and personal development and that the following proficiencies are essential. Children should be able to:

- recall and give details of past experiences
- reason about present and remembered experiences
- anticipate future events and predict the outcome
- recognise and offer solutions to problems
- plan and survey alternatives from possible courses of action
- project into the experiences and feelings of others
- use imagination to build scenes through the use of language

Process drama puts children into fictional situations in which they need to use language for each of those purposes. Parsons, Schaffner, Little and Felton (1984) compared the language used in process drama lessons (defined as 'being and doing within an imaginary situation') with language used in a control sample of non-drama lessons. Drama forms such as dance, story-building, the speaking of poetry and the development and use of scripts were omitted but the development of presentational drama, that is drama which is to be shown, was included. Their findings suggested that process drama, (but not presentational drama) encouraged children to use higher abstractional discourse than was the case in non drama classrooms.

Parsons (1991, p.100) believes that effective questioning in a drama experience

> *helps establish the fictional context, moves the drama along, challenges children's assumptions and draws from them language that expresses their deepest level of thought and feeling ... increases children's awareness of social behaviour, moral responsibilities and actions and broadens their own thinking, attitudes and understanding*

'I'm not sure why pterodactyls have eggs,' said in a wondering tone, is a more empowering questions than asking firmly 'Now what are pterodactyl's eggs for?' Questions that ask 'why', provided they are not asked in a challenging tone when they can communicate 'disapproval, disbelief and distrust' (Stewart and Cash, 1988 p.66) are 'the great educational questions that guide discovery.' (Morgan and Saxton, 1991 p.69) and encourage children to speculate, predict and theorise. 'Why were Cinderella's stepsisters so mean to her?' 'Why didn't her father stop them?' 'Why did the magic stop at midnight?'

Questions which ask 'what might happen if?' encourage children to imagine and suggest alternative paths for the drama, possible solutions to problems that arise and ways of avoiding unwanted consequences. In s drama in which the children were travelling towards an unknown destination, the teacher asked, 'I wonder what will happen if we come to something we can't get past?' The answers to such a question can provide the content for the next part of the drama.

Perhaps the children might suggest such a challenge or the teacher could continue, 'Shall we see? What shall we say will happen on our journey that might cause us problems?' This is where planning within the experience comes in. If the children suggest a physical difficulty (a river full of crocodiles, perhaps) then teacher and children can work out and enact the solution. If they suggest meeting someone or something that opposes them in their task, the teacher (or another adult) can take that role, building the character from the children's ideas as was suggested in Chapter Two. If the character is portrayed as a pathetic creature the children will have a different set of problems to deal with than if it is fierce. In either case, the predicament confronting the children can be challenging. Perhaps this creature has been told to guard the area and will be in trouble if it allows the group to pass; perhaps it is lost and starving itself; perhaps it is there to save travellers from an even worse dilemma which will they will meet if they go further. Some of these ideas may have been thought of by the teacher as he or she planned the experience; some might emanate from suggestions made by the children.

Empowering questions are often phrased as statements which invite children to think about an issue. Here are some examples.

- She says she needs shoes that will take her a long way.
- I wonder what makes someone steal things.
- I wish I knew how we could cross that river.
- I don't know what we should do next.
- I often wonder what would happen if there were no more trees.

The way in which the questions are asked is vital. Good drama questions do not confront children but encourage children and teacher to explore the issues together. Morgan and Saxton (1991a p.12-15) believe questions can be used for a variety of purposes. The examples are from a lesson on the migratory patterns of birds undertaken with a class of five-year-olds in Dublin.

- to explore the understanding of an issue (I wonder why this bird looks so sad)
- to examine children's application of what they know (Well if its family has flown south for the winter, where would they have gone, do you think?)
- to ask them to support their arguments (But why do birds need to leave Dublin just because it is cold?)
- to reflect on their ideas and their practices (How could we take this bird from Dublin to Portugal? How are we going to look after it while we are on the way?)

- to defend their beliefs (Well, now we are in Portugal, how will we ever find its family?)

Responding

The dialogue of questioning has two aspects; the posing of the question and the reaction to the children's responses. Children are empowered when their suggestions are taken seriously. Fewer questions may be better than many. Wood's (1986 p.207) research suggested that when teachers asked fewer questions, children answered more fully, using their developing language to share their ideas and understanding. Rowe (1986) discovered that the length and complexity of children's answers to teachers' questions increase dramatically when teachers are willing to wait just a few seconds after they ask a question. The children give longer answers, more children are likely to respond, the responses given are more analytical, creative and evaluative and the lessons themselves are perceived by the children as being more interesting (Morgan and Saxton, 1991).

Sometimes teachers are so relieved that a response has been made that they barely allow a child to finish before asking another question or making a comment, beginning their response less that a second after the child has spoken. If teachers wait three seconds or more after a child has finished speaking, Rowe (1986) discovered, children give longer responses with pronounced changes in the use of language and logic. They are more likely to make inferences that are supported by evidence and logical argument, exchanges between children increase, more children participate in discussions, failure to respond decreases and so do disciplinary problems. As one child was reported to have said to his mother, 'It's the first time in all my years at school that anybody cared about what I really thought- not just what I am supposed to say.'

All contributions should be acknowledged as intelligent and potentially useful contributions to the discussion. This can be done by repeating what the children have said in a voice that indicates it was an impressive suggestion to have made. With small children a respectful repetition testifies that the child's idea was valued; it was worth repeating. The teacher may choose to upgrade the language, but there is a danger that young children, especially those with language difficulties, will not recognise the upgraded repetition as their contribution and may well think that what they said was ignored.

Another advantage of repeating children's responses is that it allows everyone else to hear what has been suggested. If the children are sitting in a gathered group in front of the teacher and several children are trying to say something, it is often hard for everyone in the group to understand what has been said. Pre-schoolers' clarity of language may be poor and so not understood by other children. A third advantage is that it ensures the teacher has heard and understood what the child has said. If misunderstood, the child has an opportunity to correct the teacher's interpretation of what was said.

However, repetition of children's responses can pose problems. Children, particularly as they become more competent in language, can feel irritated if their words are repeated by the teacher and less likely to contribute further. By using the techniques of active listening, the teacher can be seen to accept and value the child's contribution, allow the other children to understand it as well and ensure that it has been understood by the teacher. A child might suggest, 'She wants something to eat,' to which an active listening response might be 'You think she might be hungry.' The teacher's paralanguage and non-verbal communication can indicate that this is an intelligent idea which merits further consideration. If children feel their ideas have been valued, they will not mind if other suggestions are, eventually, acted upon.

It is not unusual for young children to be slow to answer the questions posed. This may be because the questions themselves are complex and demand thought. 'How many days in a week?' requires less thought than 'I wonder why there are *seven* days in a week.' If the children are new to process drama they may not be sure about what is happening and so not confident enough, at the beginning of the lesson, to make suggestions.

When teachers' questions are greeted with silence they may be tempted to answer the questions themselves. This will prove to be counterproductive. Children quickly learn that if they do not answer teachers' questions, teachers will answer themselves and so the children have only to wait in silence for a minute or two before the teacher comes forward with an idea. If teachers ask as if they really want to know, waiting for answers makes sense. A teacher describes her own experience with the under-threes:

> *It really takes a lot to get them to be confident in their own ideas. They want me to say it but I'm always the person who doesn't know and I've learnt that if I don't know it then I can't come up with the answer. Sometimes...in the past, I would ask them a question and then if no-one answered, I would say the answer. Then they would expect it, so if you don't know it, you have to not know it and you don't know it all the way through.*
>
> (Gates, 1996).

Children need time to think and search their minds for related information they can bring to bear on the problem. If teachers can keep this in mind when a question is met by silence, it is less likely to be such an un-nerving experience. Children might be silent because they are *thinking* and need time to formulate their ideas. Waiting for the children's responses empowers children for it suggests their responses are worth waiting for. Children are likely to be committed to their own decisions and suggestions while they may or may not feel any commitment to the teacher's ideas. Waiting for children to respond is time well spent.

Sometimes the teacher will feel tempted to rephrase the question. This can serve to clarify the issue but it can also confuse. While the children are thinking about the question that has been posed, another is asked before they have a chance to answer the first one and the children may not be clear which one they should be addressing. It may appear to the teacher that the same question is being asked in a slightly different way. For children, especially children who have difficulties with language, it may seem as if the teacher has moved on to something entirely different.

How long does the teacher have to wait and is there anything that can be done while waiting? It is important to recognise that the wait might only be fifteen seconds after the question is asked, but if teachers are used to waiting one second or less (Rowe, 1986) this can seem like an eternity. The teacher, assuming a wondering expression, can afford to sit in silence. If necessary the question can be repeated after a time. Eventually, a response will come that the teacher can use.

Children with limited verbal abilities (children under three, children who are not yet proficient in English, although they may be competent in another language or children with some developmental delay) might be particularly slow to respond. Waiting for a response is as important with these children as it is with any other group.

I was working with a group of severely developmentally delayed five and six-year-olds. Their teacher was in role as a fairy, costumed in a long dress, a tiara and wings. She had donned the costume in front of the group who then left the space. I explained that when we came back, this person would no longer be their teacher but would be someone special in the drama. On their return, they found her asleep on a chair.

My aim was to get the children to respond to the fairy in some way and I began with some wondering remarks interspersed with periods of silence as the children looked at the character. 'I wonder what she is doing there?' Eventually, a little boy who had no speech and was strapped into a standing frame made some sounds. I did not think these sounds were deliberate but knew they provided a response with which I could work to extend the drama.

'Daniel thinks we should speak to her'. I repeated the sounds he made, making them purposeful rather than random. Daniel looked pleased and clapped his hands. This provided another response I could use. 'Daniel thinks we should clap our hands'. I did so, so did the other carers and so did some of the children. I gave the fairy a verbal signal (as discussed in Chapter Two) to wake up, which she did, very slowly, and the drama proceeded. (The plan for this drama is in Chapter Eight).

WITHHOLDING EXPERTISE

Chapter Two stressed the importance of casting children in roles in which they assume the expertise needed for the resolution of the problems to be posed in the drama. The consequences of using appropriate language registers and empowering questioning techniques have been emphasised. Through the use of these strategies, teachers can develop the ability to withhold their own expertise and so signal to the group that it is their ideas and not those of the teacher, that will make the drama work (Wagner, 1976 p.97). Even those suggestions that seem (to the teacher) far-fetched, improbable, silly or in an adult's opinion, wrong, can be accepted. If it is evident that the children are not in possession of some vital piece of information, they need not be corrected. Children will quickly sense that the teacher believes there are right and wrong answers to the questions asked of them. Morgan and Saxton (1991a, p.13) point out that it is easy to have a facial expression or tone of voice that gives messages to the group. Children want to please and they watch teachers closely for signs of approval or disapproval. These observations may encourage children to answer because they believe they are giving the teacher what is wanted or they may refrain from answering because they feel teacher disapproval of their ideas.

If the children are asked 'What are monsters like?' the response might be 'They are huge and very frightening'. It may be tempting to smile approvingly at such an explanation but it is probably better to look serious and a little worried and say something like 'Are they?'. The way is left open for further contributions from the children.

If a child responded to the question, 'I wonder why the first little pig built his house of straw' by saying, 'Because he thought it would be strong' the teacher's response might be another question asked in perfect seriousness. 'Why would he think that, I wonder?' When asking some agricultural advisers (children in role) about certain animals on their farm one boy assured me that water buffalos gave water. No-one disagreed and as the misinformation was not going to affect the direction the drama was likely to take, I decided to let the statement stand. There will be other opportunities in another class time to clarify the situation if the teacher believes it is necessary to do so.

When teachers withhold their expertise they do not nullify their positions as leaders or facilitators of the drama; far from it. As Booth (1997) has phrased it, 'The teacher is driving the bus.' Teachers monitor the quality of the experience, sharing the power with the children in an alliance which allows the group to achieve in ways that would not be possible if the traditional pedagogic relationship was followed with power flowing from teachers (who knows the most) to the children (who know the least) (Rabinov, 1984 p.378). In process drama a bond develops as teachers and children form an association of artist companions (Tandy, 1993 p.5), working towards a collective goal.

Delaying into experience

The willingness of teachers to withhold their own expertise, leads to another feature of a successful drama experience, the ability of the teacher to work slowly. Davies claims (1983 p.58) that, left to themselves, children will 'run through War and Peace, Ben Hur and all the stories of the Brothers Grimm in five minutes flat'. The teacher's role is to encourage children to reflect and consider the implications of their decisions and this takes time. Obviously, effective questioning is important. So too is the teacher's ability to hold children back from reaching instant solutions.

When a problem arises in drama it is not unusual for young children to come up with quick and often simplistic answers. Good drama is not achieved by accepting instant solutions. It is built slowly by encouraging children to consider a number of possibilities before deciding on a course of action. There are several techniques to slow the drama and to help children work through the problems posed in more depth.

If the problem posed is one of loss, such as that posed in a drama in which a dinosaur lost her egg, there is a risk that the children will 'find' it immediately. This can be forestalled by the teacher in role indicating, as the problem is introduced, that the egg was lost 'a long way from here'. If a child does produce an instant egg, it is possible for the dinosaur to examine it and to indicate verbally or non-verbally, that this is not the one she lost. There is a danger that all the children will 'find' eggs the dinosaur must examine and reject and this should be avoided. It can lead to an unproductive episode which seems as if it will never end as children 'find' more and more eggs. It is quite possible for the teacher/facilitator to come out of role and say, 'You know, we'll have a better drama if we say that this dinosaur lost her egg a long way from here and we have to travel there before we can find it. Where shall we say she lost that egg?' This question puts the ball back into the children's court. They are given an opportunity to consider how the drama should proceed. Their suggestions can be accepted, discussed and decided upon. It is usually possible to combine several suggestions as the journey is planned.

When a drama has progressed to the point where a solution to the problem is imminent, delaying tactics can again be useful. This prevents children fastening onto a simplistic answer to a complex problem and forces them to consider alternative possibilities. On one occasion, in the dinosaur drama, the children had decided the egg had been stolen by a brontosaurus. Another adult assumed this role, (having been coached in proper brontosaurus movement and sounds by the group, a delaying tactic in itself) and was found in a cave (again the children's idea) guarding the stolen egg. The children wanted to descend on the thief and reclaim the egg for the tyrannosaurus with whom they had now bonded. The tyrannosaurus shook her head and indicated, non-verbally, that would be disastrous. The teacher/facilitator sat down with the group and asked why the owner of the egg was so distressed. A child said, 'She is frightened that the egg might get broken'. The tyrannosaurus nodded convincingly and the group realised they must consider alternative solutions that would protect the egg and at the same time, return it to its rightful owner.

There are other techniques to help slow the action that teachers can add to their repertoires. Davies (1983, p. 59) refers to 'the inspection'. If the children are in role as firefighters and are all set to fight a fire, the teacher, in role as an inspector of firefighters can delay their headlong rush by insisting on inspecting them all to make sure they are properly dressed. 'Have you all got your helmets on? Your boots? Your coats? Your pants?' Then the 'inspector' can walk slowly round the group, 'checking' they are all fully prepared. An addition to this technique can be introduced after the new character has entered. Out of role the teacher can say, 'Who do you think that person was?' and listen to the children's ideas. 'When that person says 'Good morning', how would the fire fighters reply?' The scene can be re-enacted using the responses suggested by the group.

If the children have decided that they will travel to their destination on a form of individual transport (motor bikes, jet fighters, helicopters, speedboats might be suggested) the 'inspection' technique can forestall wild and aimless tearing around the room. 'You've all got motor bikes, have you? Well I don't want to set off with people who are dangerous riders. What do you wear when you ride your motor bikes?' Usually the children will tell of relevant clothing and equipment. If the teacher wants to extend their thinking, further questions could be asked: 'What do you wear on your feet? The teacher can insist that they don all this clothing and the group can be inspected as in the previous example. Then the teacher can say 'Just wheel your motor bikes out here. Are you all careful riders?' They are. 'Well, show me. Get on your bikes and ride up to the end of the street. Hmmm, that looks all right. Now ride back down here. Now ride around in a circle. Turn around and ride round the other way. Now when I say stop, let me see if your brakes work.' As well as being a bit of fun for the children and getting them up and moving, this sort of activity slows the drama down, and ensures that the children will not behave wildly when the actual enactment begins. They will have got it out of their systems before they start.

Another technique (Davies, 1983 p.59) is 'the demonstration'. Its use in enabling children to coach an adult who is to take a role in the drama has been discussed in Chapter Two. It can also be used when the children have suggested they travel somewhere in a bus, aeroplane, ship, submarine or any other form of group transport. The teacher (or another adult) can take the role of the driver/pilot/captain, but has no experience in driving this form of transport. The children can be asked to demonstrate. The driver is then asked to park the vehicle in a designated place, the group can climb aboard and the journey can begin. It might be necessary to say 'If this was a real bus, everyone would sit down, but as it is a drama bus we will all have to stand up so we can move with the bus.'

Another way of slowing the action is to encourage each child to contribute some information about an event in the drama. Perhaps the teacher and children are in role as pirates and everyone has dug up some buried treasure. The group sit in a circle with their 'treasure' in front of them and describe what they have found. Some children will be imaginative and original in their description, others will repeat what someone else said, while a few will mention something not usually thought of as treasure. Amazement at the variety of treasure the pirates have unearthed can be expressed or amazement that everyone seems to have found the same sorts of things

RITUAL AND CEREMONY

The use of ritual and ceremony are vital constituents of the theatre and are similarly significant in process drama. Children experience rituals and ceremonies on a regular basis for they are a part of human experience and provide ways 'of understanding and celebrating our own lives in the context of our communities' (O'Neill, 1995 p.147). Children and their families may have rituals and ceremonies associated with meals, bedtimes, holidays, social festivals, family get-togethers, and religious events. Schools also have rituals and ceremonies.

Within a drama experience they can be 'a form of voluntary compulsion' (O"Toole, 1992 p.160) which can slow the drama, giving the children an opportunity to reflect on what is happening. At the same time, they are being engaged in a forceful dramatic experience which can help the group bind meaning together by using a technique with which they are already familiar. A ritual, which is usually repetitious, should be presented and enacted as the serious undertaking it is. If the teacher treats it as important, the children do, too.

In the drama about the migration of birds (already referred to and given in detail in Chapter Eight) a class decided they would travel by boat to Portugal which, they concluded, was the country to which the lost bird's family had flown. The group used a table and two chairs to construct the gangway. The teacher took the role of ship's captain, explaining that as each person boarded the ship he/she must salute and say, "Aye Aye Captain". In a drama in which the group were cast as chefs who were to prepare Cinderella's marriage feast, each chef had to approach the King and Queen, (two adults in role), seeking permission to prepare a particular dish. The King or Queen repeated the suggestion and nodded regally, saying, 'That is satisfactory.'

Alternatively, the children may have to consider the best way to effect an important happening. 'What do we have to do to get the creature to appear?' The children's suggestions can be accepted and adapted to form a ritual or ceremony in which all must take part. The activity can be as simple as children clapping their hands and turning around three times. Children might suggest some action or gesture. Perhaps some special words must be spoken.

A ritual can be simple or elaborate but it is always unhurried. If the teacher wants to develop a ritual further it is easy to do so by ensuring that the next step in the drama does not take place while it remains simple. The children's thinking can be extended by asking questions, expressing doubt or by putting obstacles in the way. 'I've heard that it takes more than that' 'Well, yes, that sounds all right, but we want to be sure. What else could we do?'

PRODUCTIVE TENSION

Chapter One referred to the ways in which the elements of drama (tension, focus, mood, contrast, symbol, space, sound and silence, stillness and movement, darkness and light) promote the power of the art form. Tension is particularly beneficial in slowing the action. Not only is it a key element, but without it there is no drama. It is the force that engages participants in the dramatic action (NSW Board of Studies, 1988 p.55).

Tension occurs in the suspense of not knowing. Whenever the children (and the teacher) can have the luxury of not knowing what will happen next, then tension will be created. Here are some of the ways this might happen:

- A situation is created where something is going to happen, but no-one knows where or when. Perhaps the teacher has planned a drama about monsters and reports to the children that there are strange footprints

leading into the woods and they don't look like the footprints of any known animal or person.
- An element of desperation is created through a limitation of something. The monster makes demands that cannot be met
- Limiting space can create tension. The group hides in a cave while the monster prowls outside. The teacher can say 'We'll just have to stay here and work out what to do next.' A sound is heard and everyone is still, not moving a muscle. Will it realise they are there or will their stillness protect them?
- Tension can be created by speaking softly. Everyone must whisper so the monster cannot hear. Allied to this is the strategy of requiring the group to carry out an activity silently, creeping past the monster's home, undetected. If this silence follows a joyous and excited entry into the woods the contrast between sound and silence is marked.
- Committing the group to a course of action and then preventing them from carrying it out will also produce tension. The children have persuaded the monster to come back with them but it changes its mind and refuses to move.
- Tension is also produced by limiting the time available for a task or decision. The monster is asleep. A bridge must be built across the river before it wakes. Another adult in role as the monster (asleep but making noises which indicate it might be waking up), can increase the tension.
- The group begins to make friends with the monster when suddenly a stranger arrives who wants to put it is a circus. The monster is terrified. The contrasting elements of darkness and light can be embodied by this manoeuvre where the friendly monster personifies light and the stranger, darkness. They can also be treated more literally. The group enters the woods and suddenly everything is dark and foreboding. The trees cut out the sun. It is unlikely that the classroom can be darkened, but the effect can be obtained by the teacher who uses narrative to describe the change 'As they went deeper into the woods, they noticed that the sun was no longer shining and all around was dark and gloomy'. The use and limitations of narrative are discussed in the following chapter.

Sometimes the tension created will be subtle, sometimes it might be quite crude but it is the emotional involvement it engenders which makes drama such a powerful medium. The children should experience real feelings through drama. To be afraid of the monster, to be angry at the stranger, to feel frustrated as they struggle with the solution to a problem, to feel a sadness when the monster leaves them are all valid human emotions. Bolton (1984) emphasises that it is more important to protect children into emotion that to shield them from it for it is through the experience of emotion that authentic learning can occur. By protecting children into emotional experiences, Bolton is referring to what Fitzgibbon (1997 p.7) has defined as emotional safety. Teachers need to construct and orchestrate drama experiences in ways that enable children to consider emotional issues in secure situations. If the children are not protected into emotion the drama may be traumatic and emotionally dangerous. If they are continually protected *from* emotion, drama experiences 'can be so cautious as to be ineffective' (Fitzgibbon, p.7).

Morgan and Saxton (1987) sum up rather neatly. They write

> *A good play makes you think or feel. A great play makes you both think AND feel. Good role drama makes you think or feel. Great role drama makes you both think and feel.*

This chapter has considered many of the underlying philosophies and practicalities of an effective process drama experience. The following chapter describes a variety of specific techniques and strategies.

CHAPTER FIVE

DIRECTING THE ACTION
TECHNIQUES AND CONVENTIONS

Varying the task

When teachers begin to work with drama they may be unsure about what they and the children can actually *do* as the lesson proceeds. This chapter introduces a variety of tasks in which the group can engage. Changing the tasks in which the children are involved as the drama progresses keeps their interest level high and prevents the drama from becoming tedious or repetitive. Teachers know that children persist with activities that intrigue them and lose interest when a task loses its appeal. I have seen children as young as three remain involved in drama for over an hour. This is much longer than conventional wisdom suggests and it is more likely to happen when the experience is structured so the children are able to perform a diversity of activities.

When children are engaged in a variety of tasks, they are able to view the situation from a variety of perspectives. Bruner (1990 p.56) writes of the ways human beings organise or frame their experiences to make sense of them. Process drama allows teachers to structure the experience so children are able to focus on what Simons calls 'manageable bits of the problem' (1991 p.27). O'Neill (1995 p.48) refers to the importance of developing the work 'in units or episodes' using 'a variety of dramatic modes and strategies'. In any drama the group should be involved in a series of tasks as they work towards its development.

Once, suggestions for drama in early childhood focussed heavily on movement but process drama reminds us that drama is primarily an intellectual and affective activity. Children are constantly engaged in discussion, problem solving and decision making. This does not imply that the experience should be static. On the contrary, enactment is essential. Chapter One listed several dramatic forms that can be included in the early childhood curriculum; circus skills, dance drama, dramatic poetry, improvisation (sometimes referred to as "creative drama") mask and mime, performance, puppetry, role play, reader's theatre and story enactment. Many of these forms can be included in a process drama experience. They will not be included for their own sake but as tasks which will further the development of the drama.

Oral Communication

Children can communicate orally with each other and with the teacher; they can explain, comment and argue. This is an essential part of a drama experience for children who are verbal, children from around three years of age. Children use language to consider events from the past and to talk about things that are not present enabling them to build imaginative worlds (Makin et al 1996 p.xxiv). It is the tool human beings use to sort out their thoughts (Bruner, 1988 p.88). Tough (1977) believes that dialogue with others is crucial for children's language development as well as for the development of their thinking. Language (the actual words spoken), paralanguage (the way those words are said) and nonverbal communication are used in drama, as in real life, to express ideas, feelings and needs (Haseman and O'Toole, 1986 p.77).

Process drama, by its very nature, involves children in discussion of the issues that arise as the drama progresses. In a drama based on Maurice Sendak's story *Where the Wild Things Are* (which appears in full in Chapter Eight), the children were met by Max's mother (teacher in role) who had gone down to check on Max's boat and found a Wild Thing curled up fast asleep. The children decided this creature should be returned to the island and then discussed the best way of doing this. All the lessons referred to in this book include oral discussion as a critical element.

Written communication

Children can communicate through the written word, reading it and writing it. Very few pre-schoolers can read or write but a development of an understanding of the power of the written word is an essential task for all children and 'reading' and 'writing' tasks can be developed to suit the age of the children concerned. This might be as simple as putting up a notice or labelling something. Children who are learning to read can be involved in more elaborate tasks. Winston (1996 p.22) described a drama with five and six-year-olds based on *The Three Little Pigs* which extended over four sessions. The children were engaged throughout the drama in reading and writing letters, shopping lists and instructions to the central character (teacher in role). Heathcote and Bolton (1994) give more elaborate examples of the use of written communication in drama experiences.

Scripting the dialogue

If children are competent in writing, they can of course be asked to write some dialogue for one or more of the characters, but the technique of oral scripting probably has more relevance to teachers of young children. In a drama in which the children (in role as a search and rescue team) found a lost baby dragon, the dialogue which took place between themselves and the dragon's mother was scripted orally. They had decided that, at first, the mother dragon would be angry with them, thinking they had kidnapped her baby. 'What will she say when she sees us arrive, do you think?' the teacher asked. The children made a suggestion 'And what would we say to that?' Another suggestion was made. 'And what will she say, then?' The first three elements of the dialogue are thereby formulated and can be enacted. The adult taking the role of the mother dragon has been given her lines and the children theirs. The teacher/facilitator may need to focus the dialogue as the scene proceeds. 'She sounds very angry. What can we say to calm her down?' This task might only involve the characters in a few dialogic exchanges before the teacher deems it necessary to move in another direction.

NARRATIVE

Narrative enables the teacher/facilitator to move the drama along. It can cover sequences that are difficult to enact, recap what has happened so far, span time, and provide an effective conclusion. Process drama does not have to be sequential although it needs internal coherence. In a novel we are used to reading 'Next morning' or even 'Three months later'. In a play we read that Act 2 begins 'a week later' and we know that, as the action proceeds, anything that has happened in the intervening period will be explained if it has relevance to the story. Narrative can serve the same purpose in process drama.

A journey can be enacted, or narrative can be used. 'So the astronauts climbed into the spaceship. A few hours later, they felt a bump and knew they had landed. When they looked out of the windows they realised they were somewhere very different to anywhere they had been before.' As soon as the narration ceases, the group moves back into the present; *now time*. The teacher in role as one of the astronauts might say 'Well this looks a very strange place. I wonder where we are.' If the response is 'We are on the moon,' the teacher, still in role can ask, 'How can you tell? I don't see any signs around telling us it is the moon.' And later, 'What should we do next?' The children's answers and suggestions drive the dramatic action further.

Narrative can be used to create atmosphere (Bolton, 1992 p.41) and as a commentary to action. 'Everything was silent. The explorers walked quietly along the path towards the cave where they knew the monster would be hiding.' O'Neill (1995 p.139) cautions that narrative should be used with care. Overuse reduces dramatic impact and destroys that 'sense of an unfolding present tense' which is the essential element of effective drama.

Visual Art

Art provides another useful task in drama. Children can draw, paint or model something themselves or they can interpret the work of others. The group can record something so it is not forgotten or so there is a record of the valuable information they have been giving an adult in role. A teacher describes her use of this technique.

A roll of paper was provided, large enough for all the children to find a place around it. The children were planning an expedition to the desert to collect lizards and snakes.

> *I was amazed at the things that came out. Some children were drawing pictures of what we'd need to take and then we elaborated that and decided we must have a map. They were doing all the bits of the map and some had places where we shouldn't camp because there were crocodiles. I've found it a very good focus for the children.*
>
> (Belcher, 1996.)

While the children are engaged in such an activity, the teacher can move around, talking to them about what they are drawing and asking naive questions. This is usually a most attractive activity for children who enjoy putting their ideas on paper. It is also an activity that gives them a sense of power. They are, after all, being given responsibility for creating part of the world.

Music and dance

Music, either instrumental or vocal, and dance have always been strongly allied with theatre and can be effectively incorporated in process drama. As in the theatre, music can be used to create atmosphere. As a scene progresses, music can provide a background or an accompaniment to action. In a drama in which a fairy danced with the children, music was played. A drama about a clown who had forgotten how to make people laugh ended with a circus parade to music from the musical *Barnum*. Both dance and music can be used as a part of a ritual or celebration. Songs can be incorporated into the action. The children found a rabbit (teacher in role) asleep and were trying to wake her. They tried a couple of songs but were unsuccessful when a child said, 'I know! We need to sing a song about a rabbit!'

PHYSICAL ENACTMENT

Drama provides ample opportunities for movement but it is movement for a purpose. Perhaps the children have suggested that their quest will take them into a cave. The 'cave' can be set up as suggested by the children. I would ask, 'Is there anything here we could use for a cave?' and listen to the ideas given. A table might be suggested. The table is put into place but it is obvious it is too small for everyone. This is presented as a problem to be solved. If necessary the teacher could say, 'I have heard that some caves are narrow at the opening but big inside. Could our cave be like that?' The children can crawl through the low and narrow opening and stand up which they reach the inner chamber. A child suggested that a journey would take the group over the rainbow. The same technique could be used or the rainbow can be completely imaginary. In either case, movement furthers the action. There will be times when dialogue is incorporated into the action but at other times, silence will be more appropriate.

TABLEAU

Fleming (1994 p.92) provides several terms for this technique. Photograph, sculpture, freeze frame, wax works, statues imply that the children are asked to make a still picture of an event. This is usually done in a group although individual tableaux are also possible. Working with American children who were familiar with the concept of bears in the wild, I asked them to show me what a bear would look like if it was standing on its hind legs and looking angry. Perhaps a photographer (teacher in role) wants to record a scene in the drama. The children are asked to show that scene and then on a given signal to freeze so the photo can be taken. This can be an effective control device, and can encourage children to focus on a particular moment. Young children may need some help with group tableaux when the technique is first introduced to them, particularly if the scene or idea to be developed is complex. As with all tasks in a drama experience, there needs to be a reason for using it that is consistent with the intentions of the drama.

COSTUMES AND PROPS

Costumes and props are usually regarded as being integral to a theatrical production. Their effectiveness in classroom drama may be more limited. Chapter Three suggests they may be useful in introducing the drama and there will certainly be occasions when a teacher decides they will make a positive contribution to the lesson but they should be used with care.

Props are rarely necessary and can interfere with the drama's progress. If children are given something to fiddle with, they will fiddle (Heathcote, 1985). If the teacher feels props are essential to the drama being planned, then how they will be used and what happens to them afterwards needs to be thought out. There are very few concrete objects that we might choose to use as props that would not better be placed with imaginary ones. There is more scope for imaginative thought and action with make-believe props and there are fewer problems with them as well.

In the drama in which the children were in role as chef's preparing Cinderella's wedding breakfast, I had an imaginary cupboard full of plates, bowls and dishes on which the food would be served. I was able to ask each chef what sort of a dish would suit his or her offering and no matter what was requested, a suitable dish was found. 'So you need a large golden dish, studded with diamonds. I have just the thing. Here you are. Be careful, won't you? It's priceless.'

Sometimes a situation will arise in the drama where the children think they have just the prop available in the room and, before the teacher is aware of what is happening they have rushed over to it. The teacher needs to move equally quickly, before the room is awash with the object, to persuade the children that imaginary props are better. The teacher can say, 'If this was a real garden shop, then we'd need real plants and garden tools to sell, but because it is a drama shop we need drama stock', and can then move directly into the present. 'I'm not sure where I should keep the pot plants … over here? Can you each pick up one of those pot plants and put in on one of those shelves. Oh, yes, that does look attractive.' A child might bring forward an object he or she thinks would be useful. I would still discourage this, pointing out that an imaginary object is always better in drama. Otherwise the children are likely to try to outdo one another as they bring across real objects or a few will fight over whatever has been found and the children will be distracted from the task at hand.

In a later chapter the use of concrete objects in a drama experience with children who have limited verbal abilities will be discussed. There are times when they serve an important and particular purpose, but in the main, they are an unnecessary encumbrance.

Costumes, similarly, have limited value. Sometimes a teacher might chose to put an adult who is in role in a simple costume that will sign who he or she is. This is particularly useful if the teacher wants the children to work out the identity of the character. Without a sign as to who it might be, the children can only make wild guesses which is not very helpful. Sign and symbol have already been identified as elements of the art form. Costume, however, does not constitute the only symbol of a role. As Morgan and Saxton (1987 p.62) point out, bearing, gesture and language are also important. If the teacher wants an adult in role as a cat, that person has only to slink around miaowing and the children will know the role being portrayed, with or without a costume. Simple costumes are as suitable as elaborate ones (a crown for royalty, long ears and a cotton-ball tail for a rabbit, a red nose for a clown).

Donning the costume in front of the children, preferably with their assistance, reinforces the fictional nature of the drama experience and allows the children to come to grips with the character with whom they are going to engage. To be confronted with an adult in an unfamiliar costume can be frightening for young children. At least show the children the costume and say 'Kim is going to put this costume on and then, in the drama Kim won't be Kim, but will be someone in our story'.

Costuming children is a hindrance to the flow of the drama and is rarely if ever advisable. As Davies (1983 p.23) points out, children can come to believe it is impossible to take on a role without costume or props. Furthermore, the children will be so taken up with fiddling with their costumes that they will not be able to put all their efforts into the important intellectual and emotional tasks of drama. In their own socio-dramatic play, children use costume and props to good effect. In planned drama experiences they can detract from rather than add to the situation.

Imaginary costumes, on the other hand, can have a great deal of value. I once put an adult into role as a pirate following the suggestions of the children. I expressed concern that he did not look like a pirate and asked the children what he should wear. I then carried over an imaginary but heavy box which I said was full of pirate clothes. One at a time, the children took an item out, identified it and handed it to the pirate who put it on.

The children can also dress for a particular task. 'I suppose you have special clothes to wear when you go to the North Pole. Do you keep them in a bag? Would you have a spare bag for me? Now what should we put on first?' As the concluding scene in the Cinderella drama, the chefs were invited to the celebrations and were taken to the palace wardrobe where they could decide what they would wear. The teacher took the role of the Mistress of the Wardrobe. 'What would you like to wear, madam? A long pink dress? I have one trimmed with silver and one with gold. Which would you prefer? Oh you want one with both silver and gold…let me see… I'm not sure if we have one…. Oh yes, here it is.'

Masks should be used with particular care. Because they alter a person's face, they can terrify young children. A teacher describes such a situation with a group of under-threes.

> *It was a story about a cat that goes into a dark, dark house, and ends up in a dark, dark cupboard and finds a box and opens it and in there is a mouse. It's a lovely book. Well, she (student) decided to wear a cat's mask. I was very iffy about it because I don't use masks, but she wanted to try it out. And, oh...the mask was terrible... they were all crying and I said, 'Take it off! take it off!' And then she felt terrible and I felt terrible and it was just before rest time and no-one wanted to go to sleep. Oh, it was awful. She did it again, the next day, without the mask and it went well.*
>
> (Gates, 1996.)

Masks the children make themselves can be effectively used. Because these masks are created by the children they have power over their construction. They can be a nuisance in that they provide something for the children to fiddle with, but are less likely to have the disastrous consequences described above.

SCENERY

Scenery in the theatre varies from minimal to elaborate. In classroom drama, like props and costumes, it can be developed by the children. It should not be built for its own sake but as an essential adjunct to the progress of the drama. Sometimes the teacher will want a structure which is to symbolise something in the drama. I find it effective to invite the children's suggestions. 'I have heard that you walk along a special sort of...thing, when you board a ship,' I say looking around vaguely. The word 'thing' is a deliberate choice; it is a precise and intended use of vagueness. It tells the children I know there is something that could be used, but gives no information about what it might be. I listen to the suggestions given, accepting one that seems practicable. If the word gangway is suggested, well and good. If not, I will work with what the children know. 'What could we use to make one. I don't think there is room for more than one person at a time on one.' This tells the group that the structure has limits. Children are practical and are likely to suggest using something appropriate, perhaps a table with a chair each end.

Several aspects of the use of symbolism 'the use of objects or persons to represent meaning beyond the literal' (NSW Board of Studies, 1998 p.56) have already been discussed in this book and children's use of symbolism in their own sociodramatic play has been considered. Children readily understand the concept. There will be times in a drama lesson when the symbol used clearly relates to what it is meant to represent. A character wearing a scarf, gold hoop ear-rings and an eye-patch will be seen by most children to represent a pirate. A shell might symbolise the beach or the sea. At other times, the teacher might want to use an ordinary object to symbolise something completely different. In this case, the children's agreement must be sought. 'Can we say this chair will be the Queen's throne?' 'I've always noticed that the door on a bus is very narrow. If we put these two blocks here, could we say that they symbolise the doorway through which we all must pass?' 'Could we use this hatstand to symbolise a tree?'

I often find myself in a situation where we need transport large enough to take us all because that is how the group has decided we should travel. It might be a bus, a spacecraft, a submarine, a boat, an aeroplane, a truck, a fire-engine; the suggestion will be relevant to the story. Children can build this vehicle out of something that is available in the room. Chairs are useful because there is normally one chair per child in a classroom. The teacher (out of role) can suggest that the structure be built out of chairs. Sit the group down and say, 'When I touch you, get a chair and put it somewhere you think would be a good place to start our submarine.' With older children the teacher can say 'When I point at you' or 'When I nod at you' which means the children must watch carefully.

The teacher can begin with a child who seems to understand what is being asked and should watch as that child gets a chair. The teacher repeats the instruction about placing the chair in a good place to start the submarine, then when it is in place, the child is asked to sit on the part of the submarine already built. The process continues as the children take turns, the first few slowly, gradually speeding up as the structure takes shape. The younger the children, the more important it is to work slowly, one at a time, enabling all the children to know what is expected and so succeed at the task. It also acts as a safety device. With seven or eight year olds it may not be necessary to go so cautiously. If the group contains children who do not understand oral instructions very well, (children whose first language is not English, for example), it is wise to let them watch for a while before they are chosen. It is worth while recognising that the structure is unlikely to resemble what it is intended to represent, particularly if the children are young. This does not matter. A line of chairs can, in terms of the drama, symbolise a boat as effectively as a more realistic construction.

If the structure is a form of transport, the teacher can ask how it can be started and the children can enact the suggestion. If someone says 'I will drive' the teacher might go along with that or say, 'Well if this was a real submarine, I suppose only one person could drive it, but because it is a drama submarine everyone can drive.'

It can be fun for the children to make the noises the transport would make, but that does not last long. There is a limit to the length of time children want to sit holding an imaginary steering wheel and going 'brrmm, brrmm, brrmm'.

Performing a scene

Sometimes the adults in role might show the children a short scene to demonstrate what has happened in the past that has lead to the present situation. In a drama in which the children were cast as detectives who had to been called to the zoo where, overnight, an elephant had gone missing, the teacher asked, 'Would you like to see what happened when we checked on the animals this morning?' In role as two zookeepers she and her assistant enacted the scene. They walked round the imaginary zoo, commenting on the welfare of various animals. 'The lions look well this morning….Ah the giraffes need more water.' One zoo keeper stopped and called, 'The elephant has disappeared.' The other replied, 'Disappeared, how can it have disappeared? You are not looking properly.' The scene continued until both were convinced the elephant was no longer there and concluded with the keepers ringing the detectives, thus bringing the action into the present. This can be an effective technique, but such scenes should not be lengthy. Process drama should actively engage children in the development of the story, not use them as an audience for extended periods.

Dealing with difficult moments

When teachers use process drama for the first time they may find themselves in agreement with Booth's (1993) statement that drama is scary. Yet when they begin, most teachers find that it need not be such a daunting prospect as they had feared. Some of the concerns referred to have been discussed in other sections of this book but it seems an appropriate time to consider some oft expressed anxieties.

Supposing nobody says anything?

Although this is a common concern, it rarely happens. Children may be slow to respond, especially if this way of working is new to them, but if teachers work slowly as the drama begins and show they are prepared to wait for the children to reply, as the lesson progresses, they will become more confident and eager to contribute.

SUPPOSING THE CHILDREN ALL TALK AT ONCE?

This is more common as the children excitedly respond to the teacher's questions. Obviously it is difficult to understand what is being said if several children are all making suggestions, but it is easily overcome using the techniques used at any other time when all the children want the teacher's attention at the same time.

The teacher can say, 'Just a minute, I can't understand what is being said when more than one person is talking,' and focus on one child at a time. 'Let's listen to Sarah first and then I'll come to you'. or 'Thomas said something that sounded important, but I couldn't quite hear what he said'. Getting the children to speak one at a time is really just an extension of the teaching skills used every day.

WHAT ABOUT THE CHILD WHO SEEMS TO HAVE ALL THE IDEAS?

In any group of children there are those who are enthusiastic responders. If the teacher is discussing a story, a picture, an event, these children always contribute to the discussion so it is not surprising that they voice their ideas in drama. Sometimes teachers are so grateful that a suggestion has been made that they look to those children for most of the ideas which will forward the course of the drama. In the early part of a lesson, this can get things moving, but the teacher needs to be continually scanning the group to be aware of others who look as if they might have something to say and to make sure they are invited to contribute.

There is a risk that the other children will get into the habit of letting a few children do all the answering for them, and this can be accentuated if, unconsciously, teachers let their eyes rest on a particular child as they finish a question. This is not restricted to drama, but it is a possible pitfall of which teachers should be aware. Other children will quickly assume that the question is being directed at that child. It can be avoided. When an eager child makes yet another suggestion, the teacher can say, 'That's an interesting idea. I wonder what other people think about it', encouraging contributions from other children without discouraging the eager ones. In process drama however, children who are usually shy or self-effacing can come into their own. I have often had this confirmed by teachers who comment that a child who has barely spoken in all the time he or she has been at the school or centre is fully involved verbally and physically.

What about when children giggle?

Children (and adults!) will often laugh self-consciously when they feel unsure of what is happening. Process drama renegotiates the relationship between teacher and children (Carroll, 1993 p.4) and these changes can, initially, concern children who are not sure how to deal with the apparent shift in power relationships and who may cover their unease with nervous laughter. A common time for this to happen is when a teacher indicates he or she is going away and will come back as a character in the drama. If the teacher takes it all seriously the children will feel it is safe to settle down and become involved in the interactions. If the giggling persists and it is obvious the teacher is not going to be able to continue, the drama needs to be stopped and the children calmed down before continuing. This is rarely necessary.

What if the children are noisy and out of hand?

There are few teachers who have never been afraid that they might lose control of a group. When early childhood teachers were asked about the hazards of using drama, this was a constant response (Warren, 1998, p.248). No lesson can proceed productively if chaos, even mini-chaos, reigns. The techniques used in drama are probably not dissimilar to those used in similar circumstances in other activities. If the children are noisy and the teacher speaks in a quiet voice, this is often sufficient. Sometimes changing the task or the focus of the drama will work, particularly if such a change unites the children as a group. Simply moving the drama along to the next phase is another possibility. Sitting the group down and using narrative to tell the next part of the story can also prove effective.

If nothing seems to have an effect, the teacher should stop the drama to regain order. 'Let's just stop the drama there, for a minute.' Mention specific children, by name if necessary, until all are attending again. The use of I-messages can help. 'When people run around the room/ scream/jump up and down, I worry that the drama is not going anywhere and what I'd like is for everyone to sit down over here and help solve this problem.' I also find it helpful to get agreement. 'So will you all agree that we won't (whatever the behaviour to which you object)?' Children are obliging and will usually agree. If the same behaviour occurs again, the children can be reminded 'Remember we agreed....'.

There may be times when nothing works and the teacher realises the lesson is lost. It is as well to stop and later consider what happened in the drama, in its planning or execution, that led to its getting out of hand. As Fleming (1994 p.61) has suggested such problems are most likely to occur in drama when teachers have not fully thought through the fundamental demands of the art form. To bring things to a close without apportioning blame is a good idea. A simple 'I think we might finish the drama there and try it again another day' is probably better than 'I'm not going on with such a disobedient lot of children.' That makes the children feel guilty or resentful or both and does nothing to assist the teacher in the next drama lesson.

How should I handle an unexpected response?

Children are both predictable and unpredictable in the suggestions they are likely to make. The more experience teachers have and the more they have been able to consider possible responses to a given situation, the less likely it is that they will be confronted with unexpected comments.

Occasionally a child will come up with what the teacher suspects could be a 'smart' remark. A useful technique is to repeat the observation with absolute seriousness, accepting it as a genuine contribution to the discussion. Following a 'clever' comment with an ingenuous question, again asked with complete sincerity, can silence the child who made it. It can also have a productive outcome. If the teacher takes it seriously it is likely that the rest of the group will do so too and it may be that what started as an irreverent comment can develop into a useful suggestion. I was working with a group in role as scientists preparing for an expedition to the North Pole. We were checking through the clothes we would need to take when one little girl giggled, 'We've forgotten our knickers.' The giggle and the non-verbal stance of the child alerted me to the fact that it was probably a statement made to test the teacher. I accepted her contribution. 'Oh, of course', I said. 'I'd almost forgotten. I should think you'd need particularly warm underwear to go to the North Pole. What would you suggest?' The ideas flowed and the drama proceeded.

Generally, however, comments that surprise teachers are made in the best of faith and the younger the child, the more likely this will be. By responding thoughtfully it is possible either to accept the child's suggestion as a reasonable comment on the situation or to incorporate it into the drama. The teacher should neither correct the child nor laugh at what might appear to be an amusing comment but which was offered as a genuine suggestion.

Occasionally a child will make a comment which alerts the teacher to an underlying predicament. The drama lesson will rarely be the time or place to give the problem the attention it calls for. In this situation, the teacher needs to keep the drama flowing while recognising that the dramatic circumstance has given a child the freedom and opportunity to disclose an underlying dilemma which may need to be dealt with at another time and place. A group of six-year-olds was hunting an escaped tiger. They had located the animal in the woods and decided to build a cage in which they would put some meat. The situation was enacted and, as the tiger drew nearer, the teacher suggested that everyone should hide where they could not be seen but from where they could watch the action. A little boy said, 'No, I am going to sit in the cage. I want the tiger to eat me. I want to commit suicide.' Wisely realising that while this statement could have serious undertones, they were not ones she could deal with at that moment, she took him by the hand and led him to her own hiding place. 'I think it would be safer to watch from here,' she said.

WHAT ABOUT GUNS AND VIOLENCE?

There is no need for teachers to be horrified when little children suggest violent retributions for evil-doers. These are developmentally appropriate responses. The teacher does not have to agree or incorporate such suggestions into the drama, however. If a child suggests that the group should hang a thief up by the heels 'until the blood runs out of his head' as a four-year-old once suggested to me, the teacher might say, in a doubtful tone, 'Well I wouldn't want to hurt him' or 'It seems a bit extreme' and wait for other suggestions.

Children often want to take guns on drama journeys particularly if it seems to them that they might encounter danger. There are several alternatives available. The teacher could agree and hope they will forget they have them and/or that no occasion will arise during the drama that would suggest their use. This is risky. It is likely that if the children have guns they will move the drama into a situation in which those guns can be used.

The teacher might discourage the taking of guns by pointing out some of the consequences that might occur. 'I'd worry about taking guns, because I've heard that all the animals in the bush are protected and you get into terrible trouble if you hurt them' or 'I wouldn't want to shoot anyone. My mother always told me you shouldn't shoot people.' Small children are at the stage of moral development that says they should not do things because someone in authority says they should not, so such explanations make sense to them. Similar objections can also be used if guns make an unexpected appearance in the drama.

The teacher could agree to the group taking their guns with them on condition the teacher (in role) holds the bullets (Pennington, 1987). The teacher can make a business of collecting them for safe keeping, justifying this action by saying, 'I will collect all the bullets and then we will know there will be no shooting unless we all decide it is essential, that it is the only way out', knowing that such an event will not arise. The bullets are collected in an imaginary bag. 'We don't want to shoot the wrong person. It's too later afterwards to change our minds.' An alternate strategy is to have the guns collected either by the teacher in role or by another character. The person who has come to check the group before their departure (described in Chapter Four under the heading 'the demonstration') might be a suitable person to effect this collection. If guns are to be taken, this authority figure can demand the children demonstrate their ability to handle guns and take them through a drill sequence, barking out orders which would put the most experienced sergeant major to shame. If the children are embarking on a journey by aeroplane, the guns can be detected as each member of the group goes through the ritual of putting hand luggage through the security scanner (Knowles, 1999). The official in charge of the X-ray scanner (adult in role) can explain that weapons are prohibited on passenger aircraft and ask that each person place the weapons detected by the scanner into a special container.

Apart from the morality of teachers agreeing with and fostering violent solutions to problems, violent solutions make for poor drama. Guns are too easy. The group creeps through the jungle. A monster approaches. Shoot the monster and the problems are over. Drama is not about easy solutions. On other occasions, shooting someone or something can be shown to cause more problems than it would solve. 'But if we shoot her, we'll never find what she's done with the treasure.'

It *is* possible to allow the children to shoot or otherwise kill a creature or person and then have to face the consequences. This is not an easy alternative for teachers nor one that should be approached lightly. I would not chose it voluntarily but if I found myself in a situation in which the class were determined to do harm and I could not dissuade them from it, I would recognise that this option was available to me.

I would not allow them to enact the killing, but would probably use narrative to describe what had happened. This might serve as an appropriate conclusion to an episode. At our next meeting I would present the children with the consequences of what they had done. If, for example, a group had insisted on killing a potentially fierce animal, a bear perhaps, I might, in the next lesson, take the role of a television producer who was making a series on the animals of the area and who had come across a litter of cubs who were close to starvation. The body of their mother had been found not far away. I would describe the situation in a way that made it clear that the dead bear was the one they had shot and the cubs had been hers. I would not accuse them of the crime. Indeed in my role as a television producer, how would I know?

The importance of protecting children into emotion has already been discussed and if a teacher selects this option, he or she is responsible not only for the success of the drama but for handling a situation with deep emotional ramifications. The ideas in the preceding paragraphs are not presented as easy ways of handling the situation. Heathcote and Bolton (1994 Ch.5) devote a chapter to the ways "scandal, disease and death" (p.83) can be approached. The examples are from lessons with children from seven to ten years of age, but they make interesting and informative reading for all teachers.

How long should a drama experience last?

There is no real answer to this. The education of young children is sometimes criticised for its fragmentary nature, but the point was made in the previous chapter that even very young children can maintain their involvement in a task that interests them for much longer than adults may give them credit for. O'Neill (1995 p.xvi) points out that process drama is not made up of a number of unrelated activities but is created through a series of logically developing episodes. This 'gradual articulation of a complex dramatic world' (O'Neill, p.xvi) means that the experience will take time. I typically work for about 20 minutes with two year olds and for 45 minutes to an hour with older children. The use of questioning, the change in tasks and the use of appropriate delaying strategies have been discussed already. When teachers are still developing their skills in the use of process drama they may find they have come to the end of an episode rather more quickly than they had intended. Provided it has been a satisfying experience for the group, this does not matter. As with many of life's tasks, practice makes perfect.

What if time runs out?

Childcare centre, preschools and schools all run to a timetable, albeit an informal one. Being only two thirds of the way through a drama when lunch arrives, or it is time to go home or some other unchangeable feature of the day occurs is not a reason to rush the drama to some sort of conclusion. The teacher can say to the children. 'Well, it looks as if we will have to stop the drama there because it is lunchtime, but tomorrow (this afternoon, next week – whatever is likely to be the case) we'll find out what happens next. So when we go on with the story we will have to start right where we are now – outside the castle getting ready to knock at the door'. At the next drama session, the teacher can begin, perhaps through narrative, to remind the children of where the group was up to, then move straight into the next part of the drama.

When time is running out, the drama should not be concluded hurriedly. It is far better to stop and continue at a later time or date when there is the opportunity to do it properly.

In summary

The principles behind process drama in early childhood together with suggestions for their effective implementation have been discussed in the preceding chapters and are summarised below:

- Decide on the topic, the focus of the drama and the roles to be taken by children and adult/s
- Introduce the concept of a fictional context
- Present the past history and the implied future
- Elicit explanations and possible solutions from the children
- Following the children's ideas, engage them in a variety of tasks as they work towards a solution
- Resolve the story, bringing it to a satisfactory conclusion.

While the principles and the practical ideas so far discussed are generally applicable to all children, differences in age and ability will influence the planning and implementation of any drama lesson. Children who are developmentally delayed, or physically or intellectually impaired pose specific challenges. So do children who are unfamiliar with the language and mainstream culture of a country. Techniques and strategies that can be employed in these circumstances will be explained and illustrated in the forthcoming chapter.

CHAPTER SIX

VARIATIONS ON A THEME

DIFFERENT STROKES FOR DIFFERENT FOLKS

Early childhood educators have long been aware of the need for young children to engage in activities which promote investigation and discovery (McNaughton, 1998 p.10). Drama can be a potent force in providing a context for such inquiry. This book has discussed, in some detail, ways in which teachers can use the art form to interest and engage children and the ideas presented have applicability across ages, abilities and social frameworks. Nevertheless specific circumstances call for some modifications in the basic techniques and strategies. Very young children, (the two-year-olds), older children (seven and eight-year-olds), children from non-English speaking backgrounds, children from other cultures (who may or may not be fluent in English) and children with special needs, present particular challenges.

THE TWO-YEAR-OLDS

Process drama has been presented as a group activity. Is it, therefore, suitable for two-year-olds? Arthur et al (1993 p.136) believe that adult-initiated small group experiences can be particularly beneficial when the teachers' observations have indicated that there are a number of children who have similar or complementary interests or needs. Young children, they believe (p.219), learn about the world through 'interactions and explorations'. If drama takes toddlers' interests and developmental level into account, it can be an enjoyable and beneficial activity for the children and their teachers.

Much of what has already been written in this book has emphasised the importance of the children's contributions, for it is these that activate the drama's course. While recognising that these early years are a time of rapid social, emotional and cognitive development in which language plays a key role, the verbal skills of two-year-olds are limited. Nevertheless, two-year-olds will respond to situations in their own way and at their own level. The teacher's task is to be aware of those responses, in whatever form they take, and to build on them.

Topic focus and role

When planning for two-year-olds, decisions on topic, focus and role need to be taken, as with older children. The topic needs to be within the understanding of these young children and must have dramatic potential. There must be a focus, a dilemma to be confronted and solved. This is not as difficult as it may seem. Two-year-olds have already learnt a lot about the world. Teachers' observations of individual children will have told them a great deal about children's needs, interests and understandings. As with older children, literature can provide useful starting points; most topics can be suitably adapted.

Teacher in role has particular applicability for two-year-olds. In fact it is difficult to imagine how a drama experience for these children could be effectively structured without its use. Role gives the topic and the problem an immediacy that is impossible to achieve in any other way. By having an adult in role (or more than one adult, if that seems appropriate to the topic and focus) a powerful drama can be introduced and developed.

As discussed in Chapter Three, the bridge between fantasy and reality is exceptionally fragile for little children and it is important for teachers to member that. Loud or frightening characters are unsuitable. Overplaying a role is counterproductive with any age group but with toddlers it can be disastrous. A gentle character is always appropriate although the character can display any emotion that is suitable to the drama and its focus.

If the emotion to be displayed is anger, for instance, it would be unwise to show absolute fury and at no time should the anger be directed at the children for this would only terrify and distress them. However, the anger can be expressed verbally with a serious, but not wrathful, expression. 'I am so cross. I left my hat here and someone has taken it.' The adult in role should present the character so the children are drawn towards him or her, (see discussion on bonding in Chapter Two) for the drama cannot develop if this does not occur.

Although using an adult in role is especially valuable when working with toddlers, it is not particularly useful, with this age group, to specify the roles the children will take. It is generally sufficient for them to be the people who are around at the time and who are presented with a problem to be solved.

The focus or dilemma presented in the drama needs to be one that children can solve through active engagement. The technique of Mantle of the Expert is appropriate when working with toddlers just as with older children. It is their expertise, their suggestions that will lead to an encompassing dramatic experience and a satisfactory conclusion. The drama is structured in ways that enable the children to forward its course.

How can children with limited verbal skills make such suggestions? Complex verbal responses are unlikely but single word responses are not unusual. Facial expressions can provide a response with which the teacher can work. The trick is to structure the experience in ways that facilitate involvement. The necessity for the teacher to be alert to any response, verbal or non-verbal, intentional or unintentional which can advance the drama was discussed in Chapter Four.

Here are some dilemmas that could form the focus of a drama with two-year-olds:

- A gardener (teacher in role) needs to put seeds into packets, ready for sale
- A fairy needs help with wings that have lost their glitter
- A dancer needs to learn a new dance
- Baa Baa Black Sheep needs help to bag her wool
- A piece of the sky has fallen down and needs some stars put back on it.

As these examples suggest, the solutions can and should involve the children in a co-operative activity in which the children are able to manipulate real objects relevant to the drama's focus. If a fairy enters with a pile of wings (one for each child and one for herself), she can present the problem. The fairies need sparkling wings. What can be done? If the adult in role as the fairy is willing to wait, it is likely that a child will give a response that can be used to forward the drama. Perhaps a child will simply repeat the word 'wings'; perhaps the fairy can use several synonyms for 'sparkling' as she presents the problem and a child may repeat or try to repeat one of those words. Perhaps a child might indicate something else in the classroom that sparkles or shines. Any of these responses can be used to extend and develop the dramatic situation.

'So you know about sparkly things,' might be the fairy's response. The children may nod, or at least look agreeable. That is enough. The fairy can then ask if they would help her sprinkle glitter on these wings. Alternately, the fairy can have one large pair of wings on which all the children can work. With some assistance, this is a task well within the capabilities of two-year-olds. The fairy can collect the wings and express her delight and gratitude. She might ask the group if they would like to sing a fairy song or dance a fairy dance and can lead them in those activities.

The ways of introducing a drama experience discussed in Chapter Three are quite appropriate for these young children. It is important to refer to the fictional nature of the drama. Even with two year olds the teacher can say 'Today we are going to do some drama and in drama we can be people who are different from the people we usually are'. This might not mean much to the average toddler, but I believe it is important to say it rather than embark on the fictional situation with no indication that it is fictional.

Similarly, it should be clear to the children that an adult in role is just that, someone they know who, for the duration of the drama, is taking a part. If the character is to don a costume this should be done in full view of the group, preferably with the children helping. The teacher can say 'Kerry is going to be someone special in our drama. We'll help you put these clothes on, Kerry, (even if the costume consists of no more than a hat) then you won't be Kerry, you'll be someone special in our drama'.

Having the adult dress, with assistance from the group, in full view of all the children is important. It helps the children develop an understanding of the fictional nature of drama as they observe the transformation of the adult into another character. They may still be wary but if the change in appearance is gradual and they are a part of it, they are more likely to accept the situation. Small children feel more confident if they can see what is happening and can come to terms with this unusual state of affairs in their own way and over a period of time. The sudden appearance of an adult, even an adult they know well, looking strangely different can be frightening to young children.

COORDINATING THE DRAMA
Questioning

The strategies and techniques discussed in the earlier chapters are equally effective when working with two-year-olds although some adaptations may be needed. It is tempting, for example, to think that the questioning techniques discussed in Chapter Four are too complex for very young children and that simple questions are more appropriate. However, if we are to encourage children's understanding and use of language and to challenge their skills of reasoning, it is never too early to start. In a way, the verbal limitations of two-year-olds can free the teacher to ask quite complex questions. The children may not have the linguistic skills to respond as older children can but that does not mean it is not worth posing the problems.

Through appropriate paralanguage and facial expressions teachers can encourage useful responses. Suppose a character (teacher in role) enters the scene with a thinly stuffed pillow. She yawns and stretches and indicates non-verbally as well as verbally that she is tired and is intending to sleep. She lies down, puts the pillow under her head, but finds it uncomfortable. She shows her pillow to the group indicating through sighs and facial expression that it is of little use.

The teacher/facilitator and the children can watch this performance. The teacher/facilitator might say, in a worried tone of voice and with an anxious face 'She seems to want something of us.' The children are likely to mirror that expression. The teacher/facilitator can say, 'It is a worry, isn't it! I wonder what she wants us to do,' watching and waiting for any responses which can be used to develop the story. A child might say 'pillow' or might simply point. The would-be sleeper can nod and hold out the pillow once more. The teacher facilitator could comment that it doesn't look very comfortable and wonder again how the group could help.

During this scene, another adult can enter with a box of stuffing (dacron perhaps) placing it to one side of the action and then exit. The teacher/facilitator can say, 'What can that be for?' again in a puzzled tone. When the children take pieces out of the box the pillow-owner can hurry over showing delight and pointing to her near-empty pillow. As children begin to put the filling in the pillow case, the teacher/facilitator follows their lead, expressing delight that they were able to work out what was required.

Delaying into experience

Allowing time for the drama to develop meaning is particularly important when working with toddlers if the experience is to be a meaningful one for the children. If they are moved quickly through the story there will be no time for them to consider and reflect on what is happening. If this new experience seems to be proceeding with one step following fast on the preceding one, they may feel threatened and opt out, refusing to cooperate. The teacher needs to build on the children's cooperation and involvement so the necessity to work slowly is even more apparent,

Most of the strategies discussed in Chapters Four and Five can be successfully adapted for two-year-olds and teachers' own knowledge of the children in their groups will assist this task. Two-year-olds are active and like to keep busy so varying the tasks that make up the drama is essential. Action is important, but teachers need not be afraid of a quieter time when questions are asked, problems are posed and when the teacher or another adult in role worries or wonders about an issue appropriate to the experience.

Using props

While imaginary props are more effective with older children, toddlers need the security of concrete objects. Arthur et al (1993 p.221) emphasise the importance of realistic props, of concrete materials rather than abstract ones. When planning a drama experience for this age group, it is advisable to consider how the manipulation of concrete objects can be incorporated into the solution of the problem that has been posed.

Toddler's attention span

At this age, children are easily distracted and their attention can be taken by something quite unrelated to the drama. Some may wander off to another activity but they are just as likely to wander back after a few minutes. It may be that even younger children are attracted to what is going on in a drama lesson and join the group. These very young children are even more likely to move in and out of the drama. Something that is going on will attract their attention but a couple of minutes later they will be off on some quest of their own. Early childhood teachers will recognise this behaviour as perfectly normal.

OLDER CHILDREN

While drama for toddlers needs particular adaptations, teachers who work with children at the upper end of what we regard as early childhood, the six, seven and eight year olds will find that the advice given in the first five chapters will work for them. The difference will be in the children's responses. As children move into the school system they are capable of more complex language use, their reasoning abilities develop and they have a more sophisticated understanding of their world

TOPIC, FOCUS AND ROLE

The principles underlying the choice of topics are the same for older children as for younger ones. Literature continues to provide useful starting points, and, as children mature, the teacher has a wider selection of literature from which to choose. Topics of interest to the group, issues currently under discussion in the classroom can be effective sources of drama as they can with younger children. Wagner (1976 p.77) refers to Heathcote's strategy of 'dropping to the universal', of encouraging children to understand that everyone has the same fears, hopes and dreams. By considering this human commonality in selecting material for drama, children can be led towards respect and acceptance of others, realising that we are more like other people than different from them.

An astronaut going into space, for example, could be seen as belonging to that group of people who, throughout history, have made journeys into the unknown, *Jack and the Beanstalk* could be seen as the story of someone who disobeyed instructions and had to face the consequences. A drama about the Olympic Games could be about people who want to do their best. The problem of drugs in sport could lead to a drama be about people who will do anything to achieve success.

DRAMATIC FORMS

The dramatic forms listed previously appear again. They are circus skills, dance drama, dramatic poetry, improvisation (sometimes referred to as "creative drama") mask and mime, performance, process drama, puppetry, role play, reader's theatre and story enactment. Teachers have a wider range of strategies on which to draw as they develop and implement effective process drama experiences. As with younger children, dramatic techniques and strategies are not included for their own sake but as an integral part of the dramatic experience.

Group improvisation

Seven and eight year olds may be able to work in small groups for short periods rather than in a large group as has been suggested for younger children. To facilitate this, the teacher needs to think through exactly what the children will be asked to do in those groups, otherwise they will fiddle around. They should not be left in their groups for long periods unless the teacher recognises that they are productively engaged.

Here are some examples:

- In a drama about a circus, the children are asked to decide on their role in the running of the circus. Preliminary discussion (with pictures as stimuli if required) can determine the chores that have to be done if the circus is to run smoothly. (It might be an idea for the teacher to say that most people do perform in a circus but they all have other responsibilities and it is these that the group is interested in at the moment). The tasks can be listed on the board with the children can selecting one that interests them. The list can be narrowed to as many tasks as there are groups.

- The teacher sends each group to its own space and asks them to set to work.
- After sixty seconds (no more) a signal is given (such as striking a tambourine) for the children to return to the teacher.
- The teacher may tell the children that they can use some of the classroom furniture to represent something they use in their work. It is necessary to be quite specific about what they may or may not use. Give a few minutes only for this task to be completed, watching carefully to see that chaos does not break out. Then strike the tambourine to bring the group together again.
- The teacher asks the children to label their equipment and makes pens, paper and sticky tape available.
- Walking around the group, the teacher asks about the scene and the work that is done there. If other adults are available, they can do the same.
- The children return to the teacher (again on the agreed signal) and are told that this time, when they return to their work, they will carry out the tasks they have to do there, and, when the signal is given, they must freeze in that position. (If the teacher feels the children are unsure of what 'freezing' implies, a couple of practice runs where they walk around the room and freeze on a given signal, will clarify the technique.)
- The teacher goes to each group and asks them to resume their work. Using a public voice, the teacher relays to the rest of the class what the group is doing. A 'public voice' implies that the teacher is speaking clearly and with sufficient volume so that all the children can hear what is being said. The teacher's description is given with a sense of occasion implying that what is being done is important. The teacher can ask two or three questions about the work and relay the answers, again using a public voice
- The group can come together and the drama continues, beginning perhaps with the teacher using narrative to make the link or going straight into role.

Mime

Mime is a sophisticated dramatic form in which nonverbal communication using the body, gesture and facial expression conveys dramatic meaning (NSW Board of Studies, 1998 p.58). Older children may be able to use it effectively and appropriately. In a drama about children's games, Morgan (1997) asked each small group to show one of the games depicted in Peter Breughel's painting "Children's

Games". (A copy of the picture was available for their perusal). The game was first shown as a still picture, then movement was added, but no dialogue. (The drama developed into a story about a museum).

When using imaginary props and scenery, mime becomes an essential element of the drama. The group might be encouraged to show their feelings without speaking. Sometimes the rationale behind the use of mime might be that a certain task has to be done in complete silence so no-one will know the group is there. When using process drama with young children mime is not used for its own sake but as movement and/or action that extends the drama's meaning.

Readers' Theatre

Although a dramatic form in its own right, Readers Theatre cam be a useful inclusion in a process drama experience. In a drama about one of the Superheroes, for example, a message could arrive for the group, in five or six envelopes, each one containing a sentence. The members of each group read the sentence aloud, then, together work out the order in which the sentences should be read so the message is clear.

Perhaps a narrative passage can be given to each small group that tells the story of the drama and this has to be performed as a record of what has occurred. In this case, the children and/or teacher can construct the story and then work on the performance. In a drama based on The Pied Piper, for example, which focused on the return of the children who had followed the Piper, it might be that the whole town (an adult or more than one adult in role) came to hear the story of the children's return to Hamelin).

Alternatively, they could establish a museum about the Pied Piper of Hamelin. This can be an effective technique of enabling children develop an understanding of a past event, real or fictional. The task given to the group is the establishment of a wax museum, so an initial task would be to devise tableaux depicting the main events and depicting (Heathcote and Bolton, 1994 p.86) facts as well as feelings. For example, one such tableau might depict the Pied Piper's arrival at the council meeting (fact). Another might depict the parents as they watched their children disappear (fact and feeling). Readers' Theatre could be introduced with the actors in each tableau reading the part of the poem that best describes the scene they are portraying.

Written communication

The inclusion of written communication in process drama has been discussed in Chapter Five. It is, of course, with older children that this strategy is of particular value. Children can write letters to a character in the drama, they can put up notices, they can write instructions and labels and of course they can write accounts of what has happened. Furthermore, they can read written material relevant to the drama

ETHNICITY AND MULTICULTURALISM

This issue has two aspects. One refers to children whose ethnic background and often, though not always, language, is different to that of the mainstream culture. The other relates to teaching children about other cultures.

If most of the children in a class are from the majority or mainstream culture and just a few are from a different ethnic group, much of what has already been discussed in this book will be pertinent. If the children are relatively fluent in English, the teacher will have fewer challenges as the drama proceeds. Care, however, needs to be taken when choices are made about topic, focus and role that the decisions made are not culturally insensitive. It may be unwise, for instance, to engage children in a drama about pirates if the group includes children whose families or cultural group might have arrived in Australia as boat people and who could have had terrible experiences with real pirates. The religions and beliefs of the children's families must also be taken into account. A drama in which the children are asked to help recover Santa Claus' lost sleigh might not be the most appropriate choice if there are children in the group who do not celebrate Christmas. While Heathcote and Bolton (1994 p.84) believe there are few topics that are categorically unsuited to drama, they do agree that some topics may be inappropriate for certain groups at certain times and that personal, professional, legal or political circumstances might exclude others.

If a few of the group lack fluency in English (or whatever the language of instruction may be), the teacher needs to take this into account as the drama proceeds. Allowing other children to model a required action, gesture or movement before asking a child who cannot speak English to carry it out has already been mentioned in Chapter Five. Incorporating tasks into the drama in which all can take part is essential, so the inclusion of episodes which engage the children in drama forms that are not wholly verbal should be considered. This does not mean that issues that arise in the drama should not be discussed. They should. It may be that ethnic aids can translate as the drama proceeds, so the children's understanding is assisted and so that any suggestions they may make in their own language can be translated for the teacher. The needs and abilities of the non-English speaking children must be taken into account. If this is not done, those children will lose interest because they cannot understand what is going on. When this happens, the group can be disrupted.

If none of the children understand or speak English, the teacher's task is a little more difficult. If the whole group and the teacher are fluent in another language, then of course that language can be used. However, it is likely that the group is comprised of children from several ethnic backgrounds and languages. Even children of the one nationality may be from diverse ethnic groups who speak different languages (Howe, 1999 p.253).

If this is the case, the suggestions made earlier in this chapter regarding the under-threes may help, although it must be remembered that the children are not toddlers and the dramas in which they are engaged should be developmentally appropriate in terms of topic and focus. The teacher and other adults may need to model what is required more precisely than is the case when working with children who are fluent in the language of instruction. Non-verbal communication, facial expression, movements and gestures on the part of the teacher are of particular importance in facilitating children's understanding of and involvement in the drama. The tasks for the children should be structured in such a way that they draw on what the children can do rather than on what they cannot, while remaining consistent to the drama's intent.

In an ethnically diverse society like Australia, teachers recognise the importance of maintaining a multicultural focus in their teaching and this is true regardless of whether the school or centre has children from minority cultures enrolled or whether the total population is drawn from the dominant culture. Howe (1999 p.235) suggests there is a tendency for early childhood educators to focus on the exotic aspects of a culture, in particular dance, costume and food, what Derman-Sparkes (1991) has called 'the tourist curriculum'. Drama can be an effective strategy in developing children's understanding of a culture, but this will not happen if the 'drama' focuses on stereotypes. Having children pretend to be people who belong to the culture being studied is rarely helpful. Eating Korean food, learning a couple of Korean songs and admiring a Korean costume may be interesting and enjoyable, but children will learn little about Korea and its people from such activities. Pretending to be Aborigines by making up a dance for a corroboree tells children nothing about what it is like to be Aboriginal in Australia today. Such activities can be divisive in that they reinforce stereotypes, they trivialise cultures and may also denigrate them.

To enable children to develop some understanding of another culture, they need to face some of the real difficulties that culture has had to face. Heathcote's oft repeated question 'What you want these children to learn?' was discussed in Chapter One and is worth considering here. If the answer relates to an understanding of the myths and legends of another culture, such stories might provide appropriate pre-texts (O'Neill, 1995) or starting points. If teachers want older children to develop knowledge and understanding of some of the problems facing contemporary Aboriginal society, then *Bringing Them Home* the report of the National Inquiry into the Separation of Aboriginal and Torres Strait Islander Children from their Families (Human Rights and Equal Opportunity Commission, 1997) has plenty of material which could be used as a stimulus.

Heathcote (1985) suggests that children may be able to develop an understanding of a culture by creating a culture. In such a drama, children can make decisions about the culture they are creating and the decisions they make will give teachers some insight into those aspects of society children see as important. If the teacher wants children to develop understanding and knowledge of a specific culture they need to consider what life is really like for members of that culture. Heathcote and Bolton (1994 Ch.7) describe the development of such drama using the technique of Mantle of the Expert (See Chapter One). Although the lesson is stipulated as being for a nine-year-old class, it could quite easily be adapted for seven and eight year olds.

Learning about other cultures is a complex proceeding involving cognitive and affective learning. It is not achieved by simplistic means.

CHILDREN WITH SPECIAL NEEDS

Developmentally appropriate practice is a key phrase in early childhood education. *Developmentally appropriate* implies (Cross, 1997 p.3) 'age appropriateness and individual appropriateness'. Age appropriate practice indicates that it is relevant to most children of a particular chronological age. Individually appropriate practice suggests children's individual abilities and circumstances are taken into account. It is this latter criterion that governs any discussion on drama for children with special needs.

The term 'special needs' is broad but it is most commonly used to refer to children who have some developmental delay or handicap, physical, social or intellectual. The differences within these groups are diverse. Physically handicapped children can be of normal intellectual ability. Intellectually delayed children need not be physically handicapped although some are. Whatever the special needs of a child may be, process drama can be an effective learning medium for it enables them to be involved in real situations which focus on their abilities rather than on what they cannot manage.

The ideas developed in the first five chapters of this book do not become irrelevant when some or all of the children in a group have special needs. On the contrary, they are adapted to suit the needs, interests and abilities of the children.

PHYSICALLY HANDICAPPED CHILDREN

Children in wheelchairs, or those whose ambulatory abilities are affected, have few restrictions when it comes to their involvement in process drama. If moving from place to place is difficult, that needs to be taken into account. If the children have decided they need to enter a cave, the teacher can ask what sort of a cave would be best and what could be used (in the classroom) that could be the entry to that cave. The ideas suggested can be accepted and acted upon with the teacher ensuring that the chosen entry is one all the children can navigate. This might be as simple as putting a rug down to mark the way in to the deep dark cave. While able-bodied children might build a bridge, physically handicapped children might form a causeway.

Rather than have the children travel to somewhere or something, the drama can be structured so the target object or character comes to them. Instead of journeying to the garden of a gardener whose plants are dying, the gardener (adult in role) can bring evidence of his or her problems to the children. The gardener can hand each child an (imaginary) piece of evidence. 'You can see the daisies have lost all their petals; I planted roses but these are pumpkin flowers; I wanted pink geraniums but they are all orange.'

Narrative can be used as it can with any group, to build tension and mood, to cover bits of the story that do not need to be enacted, as a commentary to action. As with any group, it should not be overused.

Heathcote (1988 p.14) refers to physically handicapped children moving in imaginary spaces, carried by the 'images in their heads'. If an adult in role says, 'Now we are up in the Tower, we've got a good view of the country. Can you look out of the window nearest you and tell me what you can see?' the children are in that tower. The fact that, in reality, they could not have got there is irrelevant. O'Neill (1995 p.151) maintains that the participants in drama can alter their status and explore alternate lives. Children can, in drama, be anyone they choose to be. The teacher's role is to ensure those opportunities are open to them.

CHILDREN WHO ARE HEARING IMPAIRED

Once more, the basic principles of drama apply. Process drama enables children to project themselves into the action (O'Neill, 1995 p.90) and this is as true of hearing impaired children as it is of any other group. In most classes of hearing impaired children there will be differences in the degree of deafness. There will be groups in which all the children have some degree of hearing impairment, while others will have hearing impaired children integrated in a mainstream class.

It is, of course, quite possible to conduct a process drama experience entirely in sign language. A more usual situation would require teacher and children to use spoken language. The use of an FM microphone by both teacher and the hearing impaired children is standard practice. Addressing children directly and speaking clearly, but without exaggerated diction, are basic proficiencies. Paralanguage, facial and bodily expression and gesture become even more important. What children cannot hear they may be able to see. O'Neill (1995 p.141) emphasises the significance of *watching* and of roles the children can take which necessitate careful watching. An example of children in role watching the action and drawing conclusions from what they have seen is given in several plans in Chapter Eight. Suggestions made earlier in this chapter that related to the use of drama with non-English speaking children can apply to deaf children as well.

The importance of eliciting children's ideas was discussed in Chapter Four. This is as important when working with children who are not orally fluent as it is when the children in the group are articulate. The teacher needs to listen and watch carefully for responses that can be used to forward the course of the drama. When teachers use children's ideas and suggestions, the children's involvement and belief in the drama grows and can provide a 'powerful incentive for speech' (Barnes, 1989 p.22). The reality and authenticity of drama initiates conditions that stimulate speech.

My experiences with deaf children have been in a preschool in which twenty-five percent of the group had some form of hearing impairment. When developing and implementing process drama experiences with these children the needs of both the hearing and deaf children had to be taken into account. By incorporating a variety of tasks into the drama, the attention and interest of all the children was maintained. By questioning individual children directly, the hearing impaired children were able to make specific and relevant responses to the problems posed.

The children were in role as shoemakers. Barnes (1998 p.23) believes that the technique of Mantle of the Expert has particular value for hearing impaired children in that it increases their confidence and sense of competence. The owner of a shoe shop (teacher in role) relayed a message from a customer who wanted shoes that would take her a long way. As the drama progressed, all the shoemakers were asked about their specific tasks. The responses from both the hearing and the deaf children were simple (red shoes, sandals, the heels) but all were able to say something that could be accepted and used. Quite often the hearing impaired children would repeat what they thought one of the others had said. The teacher in role might respond, 'Red shoes must be very popular. I expect they come in all styles', nodding as the question was asked. Recognising this as a statement with which they could agree, the child would nod back and smile As the children told of their specialities, they were asked to go to their work benches in the factory and show what they actually did. By starting the procedure with hearing children, the hearing impaired children quickly understood what was required of them

The children's teacher felt that the fact that process drama was language based was of immense value to the hearing impaired children. She referred to the receptive use of language whereby the children were able to understand what was happening. In addition, she believed that drama gave the children opportunities to express their desires and intentions, even if the question, asked by the teacher in role as a sales person, had been as simple as 'What colour paint would you like, madam?' Furthermore, they were never put in a failing position. The demands made of them, the questions asked, always enabled them to make a successful response.

The cooperative nature of a process drama experience, the sense of 'shared understanding' (Barnes, 1998 p.25) in which children and adult/s work together was also seen, as having particular advantages for the hearing impaired children who, their teacher believed, were often regarded as being separate and different. In drama they were always part of the group that was solving the problems and making the decisions which would forward the drama's course (Warren, 1995 p.37).

CHILDREN WITH VISUAL IMPAIRMENT

The term 'visual impairment' covers a range of disabilities with one Australian report suggesting that well over half blind or partially blind children have other serious disabilities (Forehan, 1991 p.11). As with all children, who have reduced opportunities for learning about the world (Forehan, p.12) drama can be a potent educational, social and cultural experience. While the basic practices of process drama apply when working with blind or partially bind children just as they do with sighted children, the concerns and abilities of the visually impaired children will influence the teachers' decisions.

Although visually impaired children are likely to be responsive to sound, they may need help in distinguishing conscious listening from hearing (Turnbull, 1988 p.70). They may have a 'limited movement vocabulary' (Lanning, 1989 p.10) and may need support in using movement effectively and in ways that are pertinent to the drama. *Mantle of the Expert* can be used effectively by casting blind children as people who, knowing what blindness is like, are well able to advise someone who has lost his or her sight. They can be called upon for expert advice when someone needs to know how to make his or her way through a dark house (tunnel, cave) with safety. Heathcote (1998) describes such a lesson. Forehan (1991 p.14) maintains there is no need to shy away from issues directly or indirectly associated with blindness. On the contrary such experiences can give visually impaired children a chance to assert themselves, practising skills and situations they might find difficult, a good preparation for times in real life when opinions and needs have to be asserted clearly and firmly (Lanning, 1989 p.10).

In a drama with sighted children many of the signs which must be read by the children are visual. These include facial expression, gesture, bodily posture, costume and props. The use of teacher in role in a drama about the migration of birds was referred to in Chapter Two when it was suggested that the lost bird did not speak, but communicated non-verbally. Visual signs are of little help to blind children for the information they need must be conveyed in ways they can understand, through sound and by kinaesthetic means. Partially sighted children, on the other hand, may benefit from the inclusion of clear visual signals.

Vocal expression and the choice of words are critical. It may be necessary for the teacher to describe a scene or character to give the children additional information. 'Oh, dear, she does look sad.' might be stating what sighted children can see for themselves. It will give blind children further material with which to work. The teacher needs to be what Forehan (1991 p.14) describes as 'a skilled audio describer', adept in using language that is non-visually referenced.

Sighted children can watch what a character is doing. Blind children might need a commentary on the action. On the other hand, they may be able to work out what is happening from sound and tactile clues. The lost bird, for example can make bird sounds to indicate its identity. It can wear feathers which blind children can stroke. Having recognised that the character is a bird and is in some sort of trouble, the children are able to move ahead by considering, as sighted children would do, the cause of the bird's distress.

Sighted children can identify a queen by the crown she is wearing. The teacher may need to say to blind children 'She's wearing a strange sort of thing on her head. If I pass it around do you think you could work out what it might be? Then we might be able to discover who she is,' and to the character. 'Come closer so we can all feel that cloak you are wearing.' If by chance the children come to a different conclusion, that may not matter. The drama may be able to proceed with a fairy just as easily as with a queen. If it cannot, the teacher can say, 'Well it is very hard to guess who someone is just from what they are wearing. You'll have to tell us something else about you.' The Queen might reply, 'Well my husband is the King and we live in a palace.' When the children have identified the character as a Queen the teacher can say to the group, 'I don't know why she didn't tell us that in the first place.' The idea is to build on what the children know and what they can do rather than involve them in a guessing game. It is the Queen who is at fault for not identifying herself, not the children.

The sense of smell can also be used. Something that has a musty smell could be introduced. 'I do wonder where this has been; it has a very old smell about it' can lead a group into a drama about an old house. Strongly scented plants can introduce a garden, medicinal smells, a hospital or medical centre.

Tableux were described in Chapter Five. While visually impaired children can build tableaux, they cannot see what they or others have built. If drama involves making, performing and appreciating (New South Wales Board of Studies, (1998 p.5) then the development of a tableau that can be appreciated by others in the group should be considered. Children can use their voices to make a sound tableau that warns of wild animals in the vicinity. They can use instruments to describe the sound of horses approaching. We know we are at a railway station because we hear announcements about train arrivals and departures.

Music can build mood, sound effect tapes can provide aural clues and can set a scene. Physical structures and objects can build the environment. An ordinary carpet can be a magic carpet. The best advice of all comes from Forehan (1991 p.14) who stresses the importance of the teacher thinking about the drama experience from the point of view of the visually impaired child. As with any drama, the emphasis should be on the children's competencies not their disabilities.

CHILDREN WITH INTELLECTUAL DELAYS

In any early childhood centre there will be children with varying abilities. Children with intellectual delay may be severely to moderately handicapped. Although some special needs children attend a 'normal' school or centre, others may be enrolled in a class or school where all the children have some or even multiple forms of developmental delay.

In either setting, teachers will find that many of the suggestions given in this chapter, and in the earlier ones will enable them to develop effective drama experiences for all children in the group, including those with intellectual delays. If all the children in the group are intellectually delayed, teachers will still find that process drama has much to offer. Their understanding and their responses will be different to normally developing children or to those who are gifted and talented, but they are much more like any other children in their responses to process drama than they are unlike them.

Heathcote (1984 p.154) emphasises the importance of epic topics rather than everyday material. The group meets a character (teacher in role) with whom they must interact and a situation arises which presents them with a problem they must solve. A clearly defined character to whom they must respond can be a seductive beginning with enormous potential, transporting children into the here and now (Peters, 1994 p.47), enabling the drama to focus immediately on relationships. This does not imply that the character should appear unannounced. Explaining that the adult will take a role in the drama and will need to wear some special clothes introduces the children to the possibility. Asking the children to hand the costume and/or props to that person who dons them in full view of the group means that the emergence of the character is less alarming. If this character needs the children's help, the group is immediately empowered.

The challenge for the teacher lies in developing a coherent series of 'as if' situations which will involve the children and extend their knowledge and understanding. Some of the suggestions for drama with two-year-olds will be useful. By scaffolding the learning experiences (Bruner, 1988 p.94) so children are presented with tasks they can manage, teachers work towards an empowerment of children no matter what their abilities may be. A concerted effort should be made to reach every child as the drama progresses (Peters, 1994 p.49). The use of props and costumes was discussed in Chapter Five where it was suggested they be used sparingly. The opposite advice pertains to drama with developmentally delayed children where they can be concrete indicators of role and situation (Peters, 1994 p.48).

In a drama with severely delayed five to six-year-olds, their teacher was dressed as a fairy (see Chapter Eight for a detailed plan of this lesson). One group decided she was a bird, which, from the point of view of the drama, did not matter. She needed them to wake her and to help her down from the table on which she was sitting. Later she wanted the children to take the instruments she had brought with her out of her bag and to play them while she danced with each child. These were tasks within the capabilities of the group. Even a severely and multiply handicapped child was able to have bells strapped round her wrist, and have her hand held by the 'fairy'. Her carer gently rocked the child's standing frame while the 'fairy' and child swayed together. The use of actual instruments added reality to the situation.

The need for teachers to listen to and observe children's responses has already been noted. Developmentally delayed children force teachers to observe even more carefully (Warren, 1997 p.30). The importance of working slowly has also been discussed in earlier chapters. It becomes even more significant when working with developmentally delayed children. Heathcote (1984 p.150) stresses the need for a slow entry into the drama and a protracted exploration of the developing circumstances. The teacher needs, says Heathcote (1984 p.155), 'high energy but slow pace.'

The ways in which process drama can facilitate children's developing language was discussed in Chapter Four where its use by teachers and children establishes the dramatic situation. Drama establishes the need to communicate in a real situation and this need is no less real when working with children whose speech is limited. Teachers may need to focus on the receptive functions of language within the authentic demands of the drama, limiting the need for children to listen to extended verbal explanations (Peters, 1994 p.47). Difficulties (real questions) are posed, verbally, but with added non-verbal cues that enable the children to understand and respond to what is being asked on them. The fairy in the drama already referred to asked for her instruments to be returned, As she did do, she smilingly held out the bag in which she had brought them. Such language as is used by the children, verbal and non-verbal should be recognised and developed.

For all children, process drama can be a liberating experience. The strategies and techniques that make for effective drama work do not change. They may need to be adapted for individual needs and abilities, but after all, isn't that what developmentally appropriate practice is all about?

CHAPTER SEVEN

ALARUMS AND EXCURSIONS

SOME SUGGESTIONS AND A FEW CAUTIONS

This chapter raises and discusses a number of issues that relate to the teaching of drama. Some have been referred to in earlier chapters and reappear here where they are considered in more detail. Strategies that have been found to be successful with young children are examined, together with suggestions for action that can forestall possible difficulties.

POPULAR CULTURE

Young children are influenced by the commercial world as older children and adults are. Crazes come and go. Characters appear on television and elsewhere. Products are heavily promoted. Rather than ignore, condemn or outlaw these passions, teachers can use them. Process drama enables children to extend their interest in and knowledge of these enthusiasms in ways that can advantage them educationally.

The superheroes and other television characters provide a rich source of material. We know from both anecdotal and research evidence (Pena, French and Holmes, 1987; Cupit, 1989; Dawkins, 1991; Gronlund,1992) that pre-schoolers are enthusiastic consumers of the superhero culture. Why is this so? Gronlund (p.21), observing the superhero play of the pre-schoolers with whom she worked, concluded 'there must be some deep-seated developmental issues the children were trying to work out'. She referred to the children's exploration of aggression, fear, hostility and a sense of safety. The power of the superheroes appears to be a major factor. It may be that the powers demonstrated by the superheroes are those the children would like to have (Warren, 1994 p.181).

If teachers decide to plan a drama experience using the superheroes as a starting point, the approach needs consideration. It is rarely helpful to cast the children as such characters. Children's own superhero play often takes this path with the children tying scarves round their shoulders and running up and down a hill shouting 'I'm Superman'. It tends to be an unproductive experience. Furthermore, superheroes (and heroines) are usually one-off and to duplicate the character twenty times is to allow the drama to lost some of its authenticity. It is more effective to have a drama in which this central character or superhero never appears.

The character can send a message

The drama might begin as if it is unrelated to the character, but at an appropriate point, a message from that character can be introduced. It can be a written message, although this is less appropriate if the children cannot read and need to have the message interpreted for them by an adult. An audio-tape overcomes that difficulty. A tape arrives from Xena the Warrior Princess whose horses have disappeared from their stables. Superman left his cape on a faraway planet and needs help in having it returned. This use of an audio-tape has been discussed in Chapter Three.

The message can be delivered by a messenger who takes no further part in the drama or by someone who accompanies the group. Being a messenger, this person need not know very much. The messenger has the status of coming from the superhero or other character, but is not an authority in his or her own right.

A drama which puts a superhero in the role of the one who needs help and the children in the roles of people who will provide that help, places the children in a more powerful position than the character and this is an attractive proposition indeed. Of course television heroes and like characters wax and wane in popularity but the ways teachers can draw on such characters need not change very much. The range of difficulties facing a character are limitless, but 'who-done-it' can be effective. The character might have lost something essential to his or her well being. Batman has lost his Batmobile or at least some vital part of it, Dorothy the Dinosaur has problems with her rose garden. The children have to decide where the lost article could be or how the damage has occurred. Was criminal activity involved? If so, who was responsible and can they be brought to justice?

Teachers commonly use literature as a basis for drama experiences but are less inclined to look to television and commercial culture for their inspiration. Yet the stories told and the characters portrayed through the electronic media which are so meaningful and so important to children can prove to be effective additions to our repertoires.

The drama space

Drama with young children does not need a dedicated space. It can be done almost anywhere. The children's regular room is an excellent place; they are used to working there and the teacher does not have to worry about getting them used to an unfamiliar area. If furniture might get in the way it can be moved, but as long as there is a reasonably clear space somewhere in the room, that is all that is needed. In a day care centre or preschool, it is rarely necessary to move anything as there is usually a space for group activities and drama is no different. In a schoolroom it may be necessary to push the desks or tables back. Even a classroom with fixed desks can be used; people work with what they have.

Sometimes teachers think it would be a good idea to use a large open space like the school hall. This can be counterproductive. Either the children are overwhelmed by the expanse and huddle together, rarely using the larger area or (and this is more probable) they respond to the larger space by running around and generally creating mayhem. The teacher has to spend time bringing the group back under control before the drama can begin and this is a poor start.

Small children feel more secure and are more able to concentrate on the task at hand if they are in surroundings familiar to them. For the same reason, I would not recommend that a drama be implemented outside; this poses unnecessary problems. If a hall is too big, there is far too much space in the great outdoors.

It is a good idea to remove or turn around any equipment or activities that the teacher thinks might distract the children from the task at hand. To begin a drama experience in a space containing a table of Lego guarantees that some children will wander off and play with it. It can be moved to a less accessible corner. There is no need to lock everything away, but it is wise to move things to less obvious positions. It is distracting to keep asking children to leave things alone. It hampers the flow of the drama and puts children in the position of being in the wrong.

THE SIZE OF THE GROUP

Student teachers often wonder about the number of children who can, effectively be involved in drama but for practising teachers it is not a question at all. Work with as many children as there are. In pre-schools and day care centres there tend to be twenty to twenty-five children in a group. In a class of 5-8 year olds, the numbers may be a little higher. Teachers who work with the under threes may have smaller groups and teachers who work with children with special needs may have as few a half a dozen children in a group. It is up to the teacher to plan the drama appropriately.

I would not recommend combining groups. To begin with it is difficult for teachers to give full attention to individual children in a large group and it is hard for all the children to contribute to the course of the drama. The talkative children can overwhelm the quieter ones. Secondly, small children work best with the group with whom they are most familiar. They can be distracted and overwhelmed if asked to work with children they barely know.

A child may take part in the drama for a while but may withdraw when something worries him/her or when interest is lost. That child will probably join in again, later on. Sometimes a child who is watching, but not taking part in the action, will still throw in a suggestion or will respond to a question. A teacher commented to me on one occasion that she thought a great advantage of drama was that the children were free to withdraw and return when they need to without anyone being concerned, as, in fact, they do in their own play.

GOING ON A JOURNEY

While journeys can be integral to a drama's progress, they are less likely to provide an effective topic in their own right. Enacting an aeroplane journey where children board the aircraft, find their seats, do up their seat belts and take their meals from a flight attendant may well be a part of a drama experience, but in itself it has no dramatic potential. Dramatic potential can be introduced, of course, if something goes wrong. Disaster movies are built on this premise. If the Titanic had not hit an iceberg, who would remember it now? Early childhood teachers may regard hi-jacks, crashes, collisions or sabotage as being developmentally inappropriate for young children but if those suggestions come from the children themselves, they can be used effectively. The teacher might use narrative to introduce the possibility of trouble. 'As the journey proceeded, it was obvious that something was wrong' and the children can be asked to suggest possibilities which can then be incorporated in the drama. This means that the children will not be asked to engage in a story that is beyond their understanding. Obviously the problems will, eventually, be overcome regardless of whether the journey is by aeroplane, bus, foot, helicopter, ship, submarine or train.

IRRELEVANT ASIDES

Small children are apt to make comments or ask questions which may seem to the teacher to be irrelevant to the task at hand. Nevertheless, they are real and genuine concerns for the child at the time and are, in a sense, a compliment to the teacher. The child has judged the teacher as being someone who is interested in what others have to say.

I had just begun a drama with some four-year-olds when a little boy commented that I must be old because I had wrinkles. I agreed. He told me his grandmother was old and she also had wrinkles. I said that I, too, had grandchildren. A short conversation ensued, now involving other children. Where were my grandchildren? Had I brought them with me? Were they in the car? What were their names? I replied that they were at home 'with their own Mummies', bringing the conversation to a close. At this point I returned to the drama. Having had their earlier concerns dealt with satisfactorily, the children were willing to move on.

Sometimes unrelated comments arise when the drama is well under way. In this case, they need not be pursued, but can be acknowledged. 'What shall we do?' I asked a group who were faced with a crisis. In between more pertinent suggestions, one child said, 'My Mummy's got a new car.' It was a logical comment for her to make. I was obviously interested in what the other children had to say, why would I not be interested in her contribution? 'Ah', I said, recognising but not reinforcing her contribution. Repeating the original question or restating some of the ideas suggested which might forward the course of the drama can refocus the group and deter further irrelevancies.

KEEP THE INPUT ACCURATE

Do be sure that the information put into a drama experience is accurate. Theatre is often thought of as having mainly to do with 'play, fiction and pretence' (Heathcote,1985) but it is much more than that. The ways in which drama holds up a mirror to society were discussed in the opening chapters of this book along with the ways in which process drama uses aspects of the art form to enable children to understand more about the world.

If children's understanding and knowledge are to grow, it is inappropriate to present them with false information. Teachers do not do this deliberately. Either they do not know the facts or they think that as it is drama, it does not matter if the material is not accurately presented, but that is not the case. When planning a drama experience, teachers need to thoroughly research the topic so everything offered to the children is authentic. When basing a drama on the Antarctic, for example, the teacher needs to be aware of the animal and plant life found there and to have some basic knowledge of the climate and the seasons. A polar bear who has lost its way is unlikely to turn up in Antarctica. If a drama is to be based on literature or television, teachers need to refresh their minds about that story, poem or program. As one pre-school teacher put it:

It's challenging for the teacher. If you are going to work in a particular area it's important to have knowledge of the subject, because if you don't know what you are talking about, how can you guide the children and give them any meaningful knowledge of the situation?

(Ashton, 1996.)

The need to accept children's contributions, accurate or not, was discussed in Chapter Four. There is a world of difference between teachers introducing inaccuracies into a drama experience because they have not researched the topic and children doing it because that is the extent of their knowledge at that time.

ETHICS AND VALUES

The standards and values incorporated into a drama experience must be recognised. Process drama allows children and teachers to reflect on the 'ethical behaviour and moral dilemmas which permeate social life' Winston, 1998 p.23), but they should be ones with which you and the centre feel comfortable. The use of violence was discussed in Chapter Five but there are other ethical issues that can arise. Children may want to take a lost animal to a zoo or circus. Is this the best solution or would it be better if the creature was returned to the wild? The thought can be introduced by the teacher in role, 'I have heard that animals are not always happy in circuses. I do want to take it somewhere it will be safe and happy.' While teachers should not 'force their ideological or ethical positions on children' (O'Toole, 1998 p.16) they still have a responsibilit to those children, to their families and to the schools in which they work.

Some centres do not like stories or characters that relate to the supernatural to be part of the experiences offered. Witches and ghosts, for example, may be regarded as having no place in the education of young children. Magic may be seen as undesirable. This is rarely a problem for teachers as they plan to use drama. I once designed a lesson where the children (six and seven year olds) were in role as Real Estate Agents while I took the role of someone who was looking for a very large house with lots of bedrooms because I had many grandchildren who would be coming to stay. Together we discussed my requirements and a suitable house was found. I wanted the group to be faced with the problem of a prior occupant who refused to move and had thought that a sad and lonely ghost might be an effective character to introduce. (Wagner, 1976 p.97 discusses a drama conducted by Heathcote which has a similar motif.)

When I realised this was not acceptable to the school, I decided to leave the decision to the children. Using narrative, I retold the story to the point of arrival at the house. Then using a voice that made it clear the prior occupant was likely to be a problem, I said, 'When they arrived at the door, they realised that someone or something was already inside'. Out of role, I asked the children who or what they would suggest. 'What shall we say was in that house?' I listened to the proposals and bypassing suggestions of witches and ghosts, which were certainly forthcoming, I selected one that seemed to have most dramatic potential. One group decided there were bombs in the house, another wanted a dinosaur to be in residence while a third decided a bird had made her nest in one of the rooms. These were ideas with which I could work, although my initial intention of having the children help a lost and lonely intruder had to be changed for the group who wanted bombs. In this case we discussed the problem and I expressed concern that we might put ourselves in danger. Eventually the bomb disposal squad (the children in role of course) was called, and they discussed and then enacted what should be done.

Young children often suggest magic as a way of overcoming difficulties that arise in the drama. Even if the centre is comfortable with the concept, magic does provide an easy way out. Wave a magic wand, sprinkle some magic dust around and the problem is solved. Process drama does not welcome instant solutions. It demands discussion, exploration and negotiation that will lead the group to satisfying dramatic results. This is not to say it has no place in early childhood drama. There may be times within a drama when magic is accepted as a useful strategy for effecting some incident that will move the drama forward but if teachers or the centres in which they work prefer to avoid magic completely, it is no great loss.

Gender equity

Drama can both reinforce and/or challenge children's understanding of gender roles and expectations (Davis, 1998). The advisability of teachers taking roles appropriate to their own gender was discussed in Chapter Three. So too was the suggestion that teachers use terminology that is not gender specific when placing children in role. This does not mean that children cannot play gender-specific roles if that is appropriate. Of course they can. It is more that teachers need to be alert for possibilities of gender bias and to guard against them. Passive or gentle characters need not be female. Powerful characters need not be male. Monsters can be female. If a (female) teacher is in role as a messenger from a superhero it is not necessary to assume a deep voice! Drama can offer opportunities for girls and boys (and men and women in drama roles) to experience a range of activities that are not gender specific (Clyde and Fleet, 1993 p.142, Nixon and Aldwinkle, 1997 p.66). Davis (1998) warns against a constant choice of themes that enhance male culture, 'pioneering brave adventures into the heart of darkness, dominance or acts of aggression'. While early childhood teachers may not see such themes are being relevant to them, themes that enhance traditionally female attributes also give messages to children. Watts (1986) believes early childhood programs often denigrate maleness. Girls' aggressive behaviour may be seen as desirable assertiveness but the same behaviour on the part of boys attracts criticism (Phillips, 1993 p.50), actively fostering a connection between maleness and undesirable behaviour. Dawkins (1990 p.1) questions whether early childhood educators are necessarily acting wisely when they express their disapproval of superhero play. The superhero characters, mostly male to be sure, are 'clearly and unambiguously good' (Phillips p.47) as they solve all problems, overcome all obstacles, are always in control, know what is right, never make a mistake and receive praise and rewards from powerful community members (Warren, 1994 p.188). Gender equity works both ways.

Reflecting on experience

Drama offers many opportunities for children to reflect on their ongoing experiences within the drama. They share and discuss the choices they make as the drama develops and consider their own reactions to the situations that arise (NSW Board of Studies, 1998 p.64). The children may want to discuss and reflect on a drama experience after it has finished and, with young children this is likely to be in informal conversations with each other, with teachers and perhaps parents. A child who appears uninvolved in a drama lesson may go home and re-enact the whole experience with dolls and soft toys or with his or her parents. At the end of a drama, children may ask 'Can we do it again?' and for some children a repeat performance serves to build their confidence in themselves and in the art form. Children love to hear familiar stories over and over again. They may also want to re-experience an exciting and challenging drama.

Children in the first years of school may be given opportunities to reflect on the drama through discussion, facilitating their use of language and developing their vocabulary. Other art forms (music, dance, visual art) might provide vehicles for reflection on the drama experience. Further research into a topic suggested by the drama could extend children's knowledge and understanding of issues that captured their interest.

As teachers reflect on their own work, they should regard what might have seemed to be an unsuccessful drama lesson as a positive learning experience. As stated in Chapter Five, however, they should not be too critical of their efforts. If some of the children were involved and interested for some of the time, then the lesson had successful moments. Small children do not pretend an interest and involvement they do not have. If most of the children were not interested in what was happening, if they wandered away, became involved in other pursuits, behaved wildly and were not engaged in the drama, then it is worth going over the lesson afterwards, trying to work out what went wrong. Was the planning detailed enough? Was the topic suitable for these children? Did the lesson have a challenging and absorbing focus? Was the teacher successful in transferring power to the children? Did the drama concept materialise into dramatic action? What did the children actually do? Was their sufficient variety in the tasks? Were their problems of discipline and control and when were these most likely to occur? What could be done next time to overcome the problems that arose?

It is worth remembering that teachers who never fail might be teachers who never try anything new. Drama is an exciting teaching/learning medium and the more teachers experiment with its use, the more skilful and effective they will become. As their proficiency and confidence in the art form grows, the more likely are they to incorporate drama into their repertoire of teaching strategies.

CHAPTER EIGHT

SCRIPT AND TEXT

SOME LESSON PLANS

These lesson plans have all been tested in the classroom. While a specific topic forms the basis for each drama lesson, all can be adapted for other subject matter. The age group with which each plan was implemented is specified, but again, there is room for variation. Each plan should be regarded as a guide rather than as a blueprint which must be followed precisely. Most plans assume that another adult it available to take a role in the drama. If the teacher is the only adult available, he/she may have to play more than one role. How this might occur is suggested on some of the plans.

The term *teacher/facilitator* is abbreviated, throughout the plans to T/F.

PLAN ONE

DRAMA ABOUT A CHARACTER WHO HAS LOST SOMETHING

> *This is a topic with unlimited variations. Any character familiar to the children can have lost something of value to it. The example given refers to The Easter Bunny. Some centres may not want to use the Easter Bunny as a symbol for Easter, but it is a character that most Australian pre-schoolers are familiar with. This lesson is particularly suited to the 3-5 age group although a drama about a character who has lost something can be developed for younger and older children.*

Topic: Drama around the theme of the Easter Bunny

Role for the children: Detectives or police officers

Role for teacher/facilitator: Someone who found a basket of eggs/Easter Bunny

Focus: The Easter Bunny has lost all its eggs

What are the learning objectives?

- Experience in the drama contexts of role, tension. situation, symbol using the drama forms of improvisation, narrative and movement

- Problem solving and decision making

- Ownership of property

Teaching/learning process

- The drama begins with the children in a gathered group or circle, whichever they are most familiar with.

- Explain that in drama we can take roles and imagine we are in other places.

  Teaching Point: *As suggested in Chapter Three, useful opening lines (for the teacher) are: 'Today we are going to do some drama, and when you do drama, you can be people who are different to the people you usually are and you can go places, without ever leaving this room.'*

- Teacher/facilitator (T/F) says that in today's drama the children will be detectives, people who are good at finding things that are lost...get agreement

  Teaching Point: *Police officers are another possible role. Their advantage lies in the fact that the children know about this role. The disadvantage may be that they are inclined to think of police officers primarily as people who shoot baddies and/or put them in prison.*

- T/F leaves the space, explaining that on her return she will not be herself but will be a character in the drama...get agreement

- T/F re-enters in role carrying a basket. The character says he/she is looking for detectives, people who know what to do when things are lost because he/she has found something but does not know who the owner might be.

- If children say they are the detectives, T/F joins them expressing relief. (If necessary repeat the definition of drama and re-iterate the agreement that the children will take the role of detectives. See Chapter Three)

- T/F shows the basket of eggs, and explains he/she found this basket but doesn't know to whom it belongs. It has some chocolate eggs in it, so it must belong to someone....listen to suggestions. If Easter Bunny is mentioned, T/F expressed doubt and says it was found hanging from the branch of a high tree. Listen to and accept any comments.

    > **Teaching Point**: *This drama is likely to be implemented in the weeks leading up to Easter so it is highly probably that the children will suggest the Easter Bunny as the owner of the basket. If they do not, it does not matter at this stage of the drama. The detectives and the person who found the basket can be equally bemused about its possible owner. If the children suggest another character as the possible owner, this does not matter, either and in fact, it may be possible to use this character as the owner.*

- T/F asks the group if they would like to see what happened when the basket was found. T/F says 'Come with me' and moves the group to another part of the room where they sit again.

    > **Teaching Point**: *As this is the first time the children have been engaged in any movement, it might be a good idea to tell them they'll have to climb a steep path, or cross a bridge. All of this can be enacted by the children who can then sit and watch a re-enactment of how the basket was found.*

    > *The re-enactment can be simple. Another adult can be the tree and can have the basket hung on his/her upstretched arm. The T/F, still in role as the person who found the basket enters the scene and suddenly 'sees' the basket hanging on the tree. The character stretches up to retrieve the basket, takes it down and looks inside to see what it holds. Don't forget to tell the person who is being the tree that they can now be themselves again. If no other person is available, just hang the basket from anything that is at hand.*

- Character who found the basket turns back to the detectives and asks how this basket could have got there? Listen to and accept idea. Express doubt when the Easter Bunny is mentioned 'Well I've never known a bunny to climb trees'…'Yes, I know they can hop, but that branch was very high'.

- Character says he/she knows you should not keep things that are not yours so brought it to the detectives because of their experience in returning lost property and would like their help to return it to its rightful owner. How can this be done? Listen to and accept ideas. Ask questions about the probable whereabouts of the Easter Bunny and how we could get there. Listen to and accept ideas.

- From the ideas suggested, one is selected and followed.

- Develop and enact the suggestions given…(See Chapters Four and Seven on journeys) Group arrive at wherever has been decided upon.

- Continuing in the present, T/F asks how they are sure this is the right destination. When convinced, T/F asks how we could find the Easter Bunny…listen to and accept ideas.

    Teaching Point: *When the group are engaged in discussing an issue it is helpful to have them sit down.*

- Using narrative (see Chapter Five) to describe how the detectives and the person who found the basket looked everywhere for the Easter Bunny, the T/F says (as part of the narrative) that suddenly they heard a strange noise. They listened again, but they knew that no bunny would make such a noise. (Out of role) T/F asks the group what sort of noise was heard and who or what shall we say was making that noise. Listen to and accept ideas.

    Teaching Point: *Be aware that the children are quite likely to suggest a noise that could be attributed to a rabbit. If this is so, the T/F (out of role) can remind them that the noise was not the sort of noise a bunny would make and can work to extend their thinking.*

- Build an oral picture of the noise-maker which is best if it can be personified.

- If appropriate, ask group if another adult could take that role. The group can coach him/her in dialogue and movement. (See Chapter Two)

    Teaching Point: *It is possible for the teacher to take this role, provided this is explained to the children, but it is probably easier if another adult can enact the part.*

- Ask detectives to hide where they can see and hear what is happening but cannot be seen or heard themselves.

    Teaching Point: *If the children want to hide in places that are unacceptable to the teacher or are causing conflicts between children just stop the drama and set limits.*

- Enter this new character who walks around saying that he/she has been watching where the Easter Bunny hides the eggs so, as soon as the Bunny thinks they are hidden, he/she can take them right away and hide them somewhere else. Then, when the Bunny goes around to deliver the eggs, they will not be where it left them! (evil laughter) Exit.

- T/F brings the group together and discusses the issue, asking how they would go about preventing this. Listen to and accept ideas.

- Enter the Easter Bunny (T/F can take this role but must explain to the children that he/she is now changing roles) Bunny is worrying about its eggs. Says 'I know where I leave all my baskets, but when I go to check, none of them are there.' Sees the group and asks them if they have seen any baskets of Easter Eggs. Expresses gratitude that one has been found, but where are the others? 'I must have hundreds of baskets ready for Easter'.

- It is probable that the children will explain what has happened to date. The Easter Bunny can be amazed and suggest they all hide again and see if the egg stealer returns.

- Repeat the scenes above in which the group hide and the egg stealers enters.

- T/F (now in role as the Easter Bunny) asks how this person can be apprehended and the eggs returned. The Easter Bunny can introduce an element of tension here, saying that Easter is getting close and it simply must find those eggs.

    Teaching Point: *If the children suggest killing or otherwise harming the thief (which is quite likely) the Easter Bunny can urge caution, for if the thief is killed or hurt it will be impossible to find what he/she has done with the eggs.*

- Listen to suggestions and move towards one that suggests trapping the thief. Enact this situation following the ideas of the children.

    Teaching Point: *While it is impossible to predict what any group will propose, common suggestions involve the use of a net or rope or the digging of a hole into which the thief will fall. Sometimes a child will describe a more complex procedure. It is up to the teacher to listen to the ideas put forward and select those which have dramatic potential and which will engage the children in enactment. It is often possible to combine a few suggestions.*

- When the thief is trapped, the group can question him/her. Take the children away from the thief and ask them how we can find out where the eggs are hidden.

    Teaching Point: *If the children question the thief, the character should, at this stage, refuse to give them the information they need.*

- Take the group away from the thief once more and ask for their opinions as to why anyone would want to steal the eggs. Listen to any suggestions. Children can be sent (individually) to ask the thief if an idea suggested is correct.

    Teaching Point: *If, for example, a child suggests the thief has taken the eggs because he/she likes chocolate, the T/F can say to that child, 'Go and ask if that is the reason he/she has stolen the eggs.' The child can ask and then report back to the group. The thief can reject a couple of suggestions.*

- The thief, in refuting the children's suggestions can say something like this: 'Anyway, you can ask all the questions you like. You'll never get me to say that I've hidden the eggs in the hollow trees.'

- If the children do not pick this up, the T/F can say, 'What did the thief say? Let's listen a moment. He/she might say it again', which, of course, the thief will do. If the children still do not pick the statement up, T/F can say "What? What did he/she say" and the thief can repeat it once more.

- T/F tells the thief to cover his/her ears and sits the children down in a group a metre or so away … T/F (still in role as the Easter Bunny) says 'There are a lot of hollow trees round here. I'd never have time to look in all of them. Do you think you could help me?'

- Send the children off to look for the eggs. When they return ask them to put the eggs into the basket. Stress the need to carry the eggs carefully and to be very gently when putting them in the basket.

    Teaching Point: *If necessary, ask the children to sit in a circle holding the eggs they found. The Easter Bunny can go to each child and ask for the eggs to be put in the basket.*

- Thief approaches looking shamefaced and apologises for the trouble he/she has caused and offers to help the Easter Bunny distribute the eggs. Bunny looks doubtful and asks the children if it should trust the thief.

    Teaching Point: *Young children are usually most willing to forgive and forget. The Easter Bunny could say it would welcome the help and the thief can be most earnest in his/her eagerness to do the right thing. If the children suggest the thief should promise to behave in future, that can be enacted.*

- Easter Bunny and the reformed thief exit.

- Teacher/facilitator sits the group down and use narrative to conclude the drama.

    This final narrative wraps up the story.

PLAN TWO

LESSON BASED ON A TRADITIONAL OR POPULAR STORY

This plan is aimed at older pre-schoolers and/or children in the first years of school, 5-6 year olds. Many traditional stories could form the basis for a drama like this one. The basic storyline involves a messenger from someone in authority who needs work done on some property. The Prince who is to marry Cinderella wants his castle renovated before the wedding; Rapunzel and her prince want Rapunzel's tower reconstructed so they can stay there sometimes, Xena the Warrior princess wants one of her castles restored. (NSW Board of Studies, 1999 p.43).

Topic: based on "The Sleeping Beauty"

Role/s for adults: messenger from the King and Queen

Role for children: architects/builders/ construction workers

Focus: reconstruction and modernisation of the castle

What are the learning objectives?

- Experience in the drama contexts of situation, role, symbol and space using the drama forms of narrative, improvisation, tableaux, movement

Teaching/learning process

- Begin with the children in a gathered group/circle. T/F explains that in drama we can take on different roles and can set the drama in different places (see previous plan).

- Show picture of a castle. Preliminary discussion of how such an old building could be maintained and modernised. Who would do such work? Listen to and accept ideas for these will suggest the role to be taken by the children (lead towards architects, builders or similar).

> **Teaching Point**: *If the children suggest workmen as people who could mend a castle, the teacher can agree, but could ask if the people who do such work have to be men? 'I have heard that women do that sort of work too' and wait for responses. If the children agree that both men and women can be 'workmen' the T/F can wonder why they are called 'workmen'. There is not need to labour the point; introducing it is sufficient. With children in the first years of school it might be possible, at a later date, to consider the use of masculine words which are assumed to include females or the use of gender specific words to describe the same occupations (eg. actor/ actress but not doctor/ doctress).*

- Ask the group if they would be willing to take such a role in the drama…get agreement.

  > **Teaching Point**: *If the teacher asks if the children would be willing to take these roles, he/she need not be surprised if some children say 'No.' This need not cause problems. It probably means they are unsure about what will be expected of them. The teacher can say, 'Could we try and see what happens?' Alternatively, teachers can tell the children that is the role they will play and then ask for their agreement.*

- T/F exits and returns in tole as someone who has been sent to find some builders/architects (see above). Express relief when the group indicate they are those people.

- T/F introduces herself as a messenger from the King and Queen who live in a large castle. The castle needs a lot of work because nothing was done for a hundred years. For some reason or another, everyone in the castle fell asleep over 100 years ago, bushes grew up round the castle and nobody knew it was there until quite recently, when a prince from another land hacked through the bushes and woke everyone up. Messenger is vague about the details…if children want to tell what happened, the messenger can be amazed, but delighted that they understand what is likely to be required.

- Messenger asks the group if they would be willing to undertake this huge task. There is to be a wedding. The young princess is to be married and the King and Queen want the castle to be fixed and modernised before the celebrations. Get agreement.

- Ask the group if they would come to the castle to see what should be done. The King and Queen have sent horses to transport the group. (They would have sent carriages, but the carriages are in worse repair than the castle.) Each member of the group mounts a horse and practices riding round at a walk, trot, gallop. Galloping may be too stressful for the horses, so we will need to travel at a trot.

- Groups are asked how many times we should ride around the room before arriving at the castle. Enact the ride and arrival. Grooms (adults in role) help the builders dismount and take the horses back to the stables.)

    Teaching Point: *If no other adults are available, the messenger can ask the group to leave the horses, 'and the grooms will take them to the stables'.*

- Builders are asked to have a look around the castle and whenever they find something that needs to be fixed or modernised, they are to come back to the messenger and tell what they saw

    Teaching Point: *Do not expect a high level of sophistication here, particularly from younger children.*

- The messenger responds to all the suggestions given, expressing relief that these builders obviously know what should be done; they know their job.

- Messenger and officials agree there is much that needs to be done, and ask the builders if they could make a plan of the work. 'Just draw a picture of any part of the castle you think needs work' or 'Just write down everything you think needs repairing'.

    Teaching Point: *This can be done in several ways according to the age and ability of the children. For children who cannot write, the record will be pictorial. If the children are able to write, then lists of needed tasks can be made. A large sheet of paper should be unrolled, and the children asked to sit on either side. Pencils, crayons, textas are provided and the group draw and/or write their ideas. Messenger (and any other adults who can be introduced as court officials) move around asking them about their suggestions. Store the plans carefully. (See Chapter Five.)*

- Set up the task. Builders are asked about the task they will start on. Send each builder to appropriate place in the room and ask them to begin work. Introduce the castle photographer (adult in role) who is going to take pictures of the work in progress. Freeze each group and take 'photos'.

    Teaching Point: *Again, do not expect a sophisticated level of enactment, especially from younger children.*

- Bring the group back into a gathered group. Use narrative to describe the work in progress and suggest that there is someone who does not want the wedding to go ahead and who, therefore, would be very likely to do something to prevent the work on the castle being finished. Ask who this person might be. Listen to and accept ideas. Select one with most dramatic potential. Ask what this person might do to stall the work. Listen to and accept ideas

    Teaching Point: *Facial and bodily expression along with appropriate paralanguage should sign to the children that this would-be saboteur is out to cause trouble.*

- Send group back to work. Use narrative to suggest it is the end of the day and everyone is tired. All the workers put their tools away, had their dinner and went to sleep. Enact the putting away of equipment. Group find a place to sleep and lie down. T/F says that while they were all asleep something happened. Get agreement that everyone slept, hearing and seeing nothing.

- Adult takes the role of the saboteur suggested above and enacts the ideas given by the group.

    Teaching Point: *This role can be taken by the same adult who played the messenger, providing this is clearly signalled to the group, or, it can be taken by another adult. If so, the children need to agree this person will take the role.*

- T/F (out of role) uses narrative to suggest that while this person was damaging the work, he/she heard the sleepers stirring as if they were about the awake and left the scene saying he/she could hear something but will return the next night.

- Enact this scene.

- Narrative and concurrent enactment. 'Next morning the builders woke up and after breakfast they went back to work.' Group returns to the workplace. 'Something had changed.'

    Teaching Point: *Tambourine can be used to bring the group back to the teacher (See Chapter Seven).*

- Messenger in role says they seem disturbed. Is anything wrong? Asks each group what has happened overnight. Listen to and accept ideas. Messenger asks who could have done this and why. (The why question is important).

- Messenger asks what can be done to stop this person doing more damage. Listen to and accept ideas. Move towards staying awake the next night and catching this person in the act (unless the children some up with a another idea).

- T/F(out of role) asks how this person can be caught and questioned. Listen to and accept ideas, selecting one that lends itself to appropriate enactment.

- When the saboteur is apprehended (following the ideas of the group) he/she can be questioned by the group. Saboteur's reasons for actions will be drawn from the children's responses to the 'why' question as above.

    Teaching Point: *Oral scripting can be used. The T/F needs to assist the children. Ask, 'What should we say to this person?' listen to and accept suggestions. And what would he/she say to that? Let's try it shall we?' The scripting can continue although the T/F may have to monitor its direction so the interchange is progressing. Three or four exchanges may be enough. Avoid a 'you did,' 'I didn't' retort, which takes the story nowhere.*

- Out of role T/F asks the group how they would like the story to end. Listen to and accept ideas and decide on a conclusion.

- Enact the conclusion suggested. Try to move towards the person being given some ongoing position in the castle, then he or she can take that role as the drama concludes.

- Use narrative to move the story to the wedding celebrations. The builders are invited and taken to the royal wardrobe where they are asked to choose what they would like to wear. All dress (in imaginary clothes).

    Teaching Point: *A court official (adult in role) takes the builders to the Royal Wardrobe. See Chapter Five)*

- Messenger tells the group they must hurry to the ballroom for the King and Queen and the Prince and Princess are about to enter.

- Messenger says 'Let the Royal Progress begin!' Out of role, ask the group to suggest a song that could be sung to mark the Royal progress.

    Teaching Point: *Any song known to the group is fine. Baa Baa Black Sheep or Twinkle Twinkle Little Star are likely suggestions from pre-schoolers. These songs can be performed with as much grandeur as any other. The important issue is the enactment of the ritual. See Chapter Four).*

- Messenger hold a child's hand and progresses regally, singing the suggested song. The rest of the group follow in pairs.

- After the Royal progress, teacher/facilitator (out of role) suggests that the King and Queen wanted to reward the builders for their hard work and ask what they might be given.

- Messenger announces there is to be a special award for the builders. Messenger, or another adult/s in role as the King and or Queen walk up the line handing whatever was suggested to each member of the group.

- Group sits and narrative concludes. 'So the wedding went ahead and they all lived happily ever afterwards.'

PLAN THREE

Topic: One of our aircraft is missing!

This drama was originally planned to extend a unit of work that had focussed on aviation. The lesson is suitable for children from four upwards but could be adapted for three-year-olds. There are opportunities for written expression for older children

As with all the drama plans in this book, the topic allows for many variations. A boat can have disappeared from a marina, a bus from a depot, toys from Santa's workshop, an animal from the Zoo. The underlying idea is the same, but the performance will be different.

Role/s for Children: Airport security

Roles for Adult/s: Worker at the airport/pilot

Focus: An aeroplane has disappeared from its hanger at the airport.

What are the learning objectives?

Experience in the drama contexts of situation, role, tension, using narrative and movement

To draw on and extend the children's knowledge and understanding of aviation through a drama that calls on and develops that knowledge and understanding, engaging them in problem solving and decision making that will determine the course of the drama.

Teaching/learning process

- Define drama by explaining to the group that they will be engaged in an imaginary situation in which they will take roles and accept that they are in places other than the classroom.

- Indicate that in today's drama they will be the airport security people who look after problems at the airport. Get agreement. Ask the children about the work and responsibilities of airport security staff.

> **Teaching Point**: *The younger the children, the less sophisticated their ideas will be. This does not matter. The teacher can ask questions which develop their understanding. 'I wonder how the airport security staff make sure the 'planes are safe when they are in the hangers'. 'I wonder how they stop people getting on the 'plane without a ticket.' 'I wonder how they know there is nothing dangerous in people's luggage'. (See Chapter Four for a discussion on questioning).*

- T/F indicates he/she will leave and on return will be someone in the drama.

- Exits and returns looking for the airport security people. Get agreement from the group that they are taking that role.

- Present the problem: This morning, the hangar was opened ready to take the plane out and it was not there. It had disappeared. Ask the security people what could have happened. Listen to and accept suggestions.

- Another adult is introduced as someone who will take the role of a pilot. Ask the group what a pilot should wear. Establish an imaginary cupboard and take uniform out and dress the pilot.

  > **Teaching Point**: *See Chapter Five for a description of this strategy*

- Ask the group what sort of an aeroplane we should say has disappeared. Get ideas and select one.

  > **Teaching Point**: *Children can only draw on what they know. If their response is simply 'a big one' the teacher can try for greater complexity. 'What sort of big one would be best, do you think?' However, if 'a big one' is the most sophisticated suggestion on offer, it is sufficient.*

- Ask where the airport security people would be on an ordinary morning at the airport, before any of the aeroplanes start to fly. Listen to and accept suggestions. Get the group to enact their suggested activities.

> **Teaching Point**: *If necessary, the teacher can draw on the ideas expressed when the work and responsibilities of aircraft security personnel were discussed. It may be wise to direct this scene (See Chapter Six for a discussion of this strategy)*

- Indicate that while they are working the T/F (in role as an airport worker) and the pilot will enter and will tell the security people that one of the aircraft is missing from its hanger. Enact this scene.

- Ask the group if they would come to the hanger and see for themselves. Establish where the hangar might be. Group go to the hangar and agree that the aircraft is missing.

- Ask group to look around and see if they can see anything in the hanger that might give them some ideas about what might have happened to the aeroplane. On their return, sit them down and ask what they found that might help us work out what happened. Listen to and accept ideas.

> **Teaching Point**: *The teacher can make it clear that it is the children who will decide where the missing aircraft has gone and/or what has happened to it. 'What shall we say has happened to the missing 'plane?' There are opportunities here for some written work. With older children, the first act of the drama can end here and the children can write an answer to this question. The teacher can collate the suggestions made and list them for discussion. It is almost always possible to incorporate several suggestions in subsequent action.*

- Agree on the path to be followed and enact that story, following the ideas presented by the children as the story unfolds.

- When the aeroplane is discovered, a problem is presented that makes its recovery difficult. Depending on the story the group have developed, this could involve confronting a thief or overcoming physical difficulties in recovering the aeroplane (it is damaged or in an awkward place where its removal would be either difficult or dangerous or both).

> **Teaching Point**: *This may have already been flagged by the children through their oral or written proposals.*

- Following the children's suggestions the difficulties are finally overcome and the aeroplane recovered and returned to its hanger, then brought out ready to fly.

- Group are thanked for their assistance and asked if they would like to fly somewhere as a reward for their hard work. Each person is issued with a ticket to fly to the destination of their choice.

- Conclude with narrative which says how much the people enjoyed their journeys.

PLAN FOUR

This lesson was originally planned for five and six year old children with severe intellectual and physical disabilities and was intended to complement their current study of the senses. It could also be used, with normally developing two and three year olds but, as it stands, lacks sufficient challenge for older children.

Topic: A visit from a fairy

Role/s for the children: People who are visited by a fairy

Role/s for teachers: Facilitator and fairy

Focus: The fairy is looking for people who will dance with her

What are the learning objectives?

Experience in the drama contexts of situation, especially the acceptance of a fictional situation, role and focus through the drama forms of narrative, movement and mime; encouraging children to be aware of the drama situation by involving them in its progress.

To reinforce children's knowledge and understanding of the senses

Teaching/learning process

- The drama begins with children in a gathered group. Teacher says that in drama we can be people who are different to the people we usually are (see previous plans).

- T/F tells the children that another adult (preferably someone they know) will be someone special in the drama. A suitable costume (dress, tiara, wings) are shown to the children who can, if possible, hand each item to the adult who dresses in front of the group.

  > **Teaching Point**: *At this stage, do not state the character's identity. If the children mention the word 'fairy' well and good. On one occasion, a child said the character was a bird and this was quite acceptable. If, by the time the character has donned the outfit, her identity has not been mentioned. T/F can say*

'Oh doesn't she make a great…um…um…fairy.' The halting speech is deliberate. It provides an opportunity for a child to define the role, but if this does not occur, the conclusion of the sentence sounds quite natural.

- T/F indicates that the group will walk go for a walk and on, when we return, the drama will have begun.

    Teaching Point: *The walk need not be a long one. The group can simply walk round the room or can walk outside and in again. Children in wheelchairs or frames can be assisted by other adults. If movement is impossible, the children can be asked to put their hands over their eyes, with the T/F and any other adults demonstrating. Obviously it does not matter if some children do not comply!*

- When the group returns, the fairy is in place, asleep, holding a large bag which will later be found to contain musical instruments

    Teaching Point: *The positioning of the fairy is at the discretion of the teacher. She should be prominently placed so all children can see her but, at this stage, cannot touch her. I chose to have the fairy on a chair that was placed on a table*

- Wait for any comments or other reactions the children might make.

    Teaching Point: *Let the children take their own time here. There may need a few minutes just to observe what is in front of them. If no reactions at all are forthcoming the T/F could say 'I wonder who that is.' The children and the T/F can walk around the character and then back the other way. The above question can be repeated, but with a sense of wonder rather than urgency.*

- Whether there have been any responses or not, the T/F can say (eventually) 'I wonder if she can see us'. Wait, as above for any reaction. If necessary, repeat the question.

    Teaching Point: *It is important to move slowly. The children should have all the time in the world to observe this character and to react in whatever ways they wish.*

- The fairy gradually opens her eyes and looks at the children, making eye contact with each member of the group. T/F repeats the question, 'I wonder if she can see us.'

- T/F picks up any response the children have made and encourages the children to make some oral overture to the fairy. This might involve repeating a word or even a sound made by the children. Fairy watches, but says nothing.

- T/F suggests we might touch the fairy and encourages the children to do that. Fairy does not react.

    Teaching Point: *This will need to be monitored to protect the adult in role as the fairy. In practice, the children are likely to be tentative and the touching is unlikely to be rough or to endanger the teacher in role's safety.*

- T/F asks the children what we should do next. If any responses are forthcoming they can be enacted. Fairy does not react.

- Fairy moves her position so the contents of the bag make some sound.

- T/F gets the children to listen. Fairy repeats the movement as above. Listen to and respond to any responses made by the children.

    Teaching Point: *Verbal two-year-olds may name a sound they can hear, or identify an instrument by its sound. T/F can express interest at this possibility.*

- Focus children's attention on the sounds from the bag. T/F can suggest they cup their ears to hear more clearly, demonstrating the action.

- T/F asks fairy to join the group. Fairy shakes her head and points to the bag. T/F asks children what this might mean, accepting and reacting to any response.

- Fairy points to the bag and then points to the children.

- Eventually, (T/F can signal to the fairy when this is to happen) the fairy opens the bag and shows its contents to the children, nodding and smiling as children look inside and begin to take the instruments out.

> **Teaching Point**: *This segment will need to be monitored by the T/F and/or other adults so each child and each adult gets an instrument. If the children are physically unable to remove an instrument, they can be assisted. If they want to take several, they can be redirected.*

- Children begin to shake/play the instruments. Taped music also plays. The fairy dances away from the group holding out her hands to the children. Stop the taped music.

- T/F asks the children what she might want. Listen to and respond to any responses or reactions. Fairy continues to stretch her hands out towards the children.

- If the children have made no such response, the T/F can wonder if the fairy wants to dance *with* them. Fairy nods and smiles.

- Group bring the fairy into their midst where she continues to dance with the children. Tapes music restarts.

  > **Teaching Point**: *If the fairy began the scene on a table, she can, at this stage, be helped down.*

- Music and dancing continue.

  > **Teaching Point**: *The T/F needs to judge how long this scene should continue. When it seems necessary to move the action along, the taped music can stop.*

- Fairy picks up her bag and goes to each child, indicating, non-verbally, that the instrument is to be returned. If a child does not place the instrument in the bag, the fairy simply takes it from him/her, smiling and nodding.

  > **Teaching Point**: *If the fairy goes first to one of the adults, that will model the required behaviour. If the group use sign language, 'Thank you' can be signed to each child.*

- When all the instruments are back in the bag, the fairy leaves waving goodbye to the children who are encouraged to wave back.

- T/F sits with the group saying that we have come to the end of the drama. The teacher who was in role as the fairy returns with the costume over her arm, puts it down out of reach of the children and rejoins the group. She and T/F talk to the children about what has happened and indicate that the fairy is now out of role and is herself once more.

    Teaching Point: *While debriefing is always necessary, it is essential that very young children and children with a developmental delay understand the fictional situation is over and that all participants are themselves once more.*

PLAN FIVE

This lesson was implemented with two classes in Ireland (4/5 year olds and 6/7 year olds) in their first years of school. The topic was chosen to complement work they had been doing on the winter migration of birds. The plan could easily be adapted to Australian conditions. Variations of the theme could relate to any creature or person losing its family and the basic plan would need few changes to make it suitable for pre-schoolers.

Topic: The winter migration of birds

Role/s for Children: Ornithologists

Role/s for Adult/s: Person who found the lost bird/ and the lost bird itself.

Focus: A young bird is lost

What are the learning objectives?

Experience in the drama contexts of situation, role, mood, tension, symbol, through the drama forms of improvisation, narrative and movement.

Draw on children's knowledge and understanding of the winter migration of birds

Caring for those in trouble

Teaching/learning process

- Ask children for their ideas about drama. (See Chapter Three). Explain that in drama we agree to take roles that are different to those we take in real life and agree also that the classroom can be elsewhere.

- Say that in our drama today, the children will take the role of ornithologists, people who know about birds. Get agreement.

- Introduce another adult, saying he/she will be in the drama too.

    Teaching Point: *At this stage, there is no need to specify the role to be taken by this person. If the children ask who this person will be, the teacher can say that will be made clear as the drama progresses. It is possible for the teacher to take this role, but* *another adult in role gives more scope to the implementation of the drama. If another adult is used, the character need not speak but should communicate non-verbally. If the teacher plays this role, he/she will need to speak when acting in a facilitator role but can use non-verbal communication when playing the bird.*

- T/F indicates he/she will leave the scene and will re-enter as another person.

    Teaching Point: *The plan continues on the assumption that another adult will play the bird.*

- T/F re-enters expressing concern. He/she is looking for some ornithologists, people who know a lot about birds.

    Teaching Point: *The character can have the word "ornithologists" on a piece of paper, explaining he/she wrote it down to be sure of finding the right people. Put the label somewhere obvious.*

- When group agree they are ornithologists, the character expresses relief. He/she explains that he/she has found a lost bird but doesn't know what to do with it. Character says it is very timid, but if the ornithologists can be very quiet, the bird might be persuaded to meet them so they can see for themselves.

- Character calls the bird, but it merely puts its head round a corner, looks afraid and draws back. Character asks the ornithologists if they could make some sounds that might encourage it. Listen to ideas and ask the group to make those sounds. Bird slowly enters the scene, looking upset and afraid.

- Character who found the bird expresses helplessness. 'You can see for yourself that it is not very happy, but I don't know what to do.' Listen to and accept ideas. As suggestions are made, the children, individually or as a group, can put that suggestion to the bird. The bird refutes any suggestions that do not relate to loss or family

    Teaching Point: *It is common for children to want to offer food and drink. This can be counter-productive and repetitive for it is hard for the children to know where to stop. Once the*

> *bird agrees it is hungry and/or thirsty the children are likely to want to keep offering it food and drink. It is better for the bird to indicate it is neither hungry nor thirsty. This forces the children to consider other possibilities.*

- When a suggestions is made that relates to loss or family, the bird nods and looks grateful, indicating that the group are beginning to understand her problem.

- Character who found the bird also looks pleased and asks the group where the bird's family might be. Bird looks downcast again. Character asks the ornithologists why this should be so. Listen to and accept ideas.

- When children suggest the bird's family may have flown to warmer climes, the bird again reacts with delight. Character asks the bird where they would have gone. Bird is downcast again.

- Character asks the ornithologists if they know where birds like this are likely to go when the weather gets cold.

- If the response is 'Where it is warmer' the character can say, 'Well, yes, I know that, but *where!*'

> **Teaching Point**: *The teacher need not be surprised if the suggestions made are unlikely to be ornithologically or geographically correct. If a child suggests, for example 'the North Pole' the T/F can say' doubtfully, 'But I always thought it was colder there than here.' Listen to the ideas given and select a place that is far away but is a reasonable suggestion, geographically; one that will pose difficulties for the group when they plan to take the bird there later in the drama.*

- Out of role, the teacher asks the group if they will agree the bird's family has gone to one of the destinations suggested. Ask them to see if the bird will agree with that as well. Naturally the bird will do so.

- Character who found the bird, turns brightly to it and says, 'Well now you know where to go, you can be off.' Bird looks dismayed again and Character asks the ornithologists what its problem is now. It knows where to go, so why is it looking so unhappy?

- Listen to suggestions. When someone suggests the bird does not know how to get to the place suggested, the bird nods vigorously. Character who found the bird looks nonplussed.

    Teaching Point: *By looking puzzled, the teacher in role as the bird's finder is, in fact, asking the question 'What shall we do next?'*

- Bird can indicate, through mime, that it would like the ornithologists to take it to wherever has been suggested. Bird-finder continues to look confused, looking to the ornithologists for clarification.

    Teaching Point: *If the group do not suggest the bird wants to be taken to wherever was decided upon, the bird finder can ask, 'Do you think it want us to go with it?' at which the bird can nod enthusiastically. It is better however, if the children suggest this themselves.*

- The bird-finder poses another problem. 'But how will we get there? We can't fly'.

- Listen to and accept ideas but put difficulties in the way if possible. For example, if the group have decided on a destination that is in another country, the teacher in role as the bird finder can say things like 'But that is a long way. You have to go over the sea'. and wait for further suggestions.

- The journey can be enacted.

    Teaching Point: *The bird finder can take another role here. For example he/she could be the captain of the ship on which they will travel and can insist that everyone salutes and says "Aye Aye Captain" as they board the ship. He/she could be the flight attendant on the plane who takes their boarding passes and checks their luggage is stowed and all are wearing seatbelts. If the journey is overland, the teacher can ask the group what sort of difficulties or dangers they might encounter and these can be enacted and overcome. (See Chapter Seven).*

- On arrival at the destination another problem can be introduced. Another character meets them (perhaps another bird, but not necessarily so.). This character asks what they want. It then agrees that, yes, the bird's family did arrive, but it chased them away. Creature exits.

> **Teaching Point**: *The identity of this character, who should be antagonistic to the group, can be decided upon by the group. The teacher (out of role) can use narrative to introduce this character. 'When the ornithologists and the bird arrived at X, they were met by a creature looking very cross.' What sort of creature shall we say it was?' Then the teacher can ask to be coached in behaviour and movement appropriate to that character. The teacher leaves the group, out of role, and returns in role and the scene is enacted as suggested above.*

- After exiting in role as the character opposed the group, the teacher can re-enters, this time as a bird, who greets the group politely and asks what they want. When they explain their purpose, this bird looks apologetic, and agrees that yes, the bird's family did arrive, but there was no room for them round there, so they had to move on. Bird 2 should say that it knows Bird 1's family is around there somewhere, but it doesn't know where they actually are.

- Bird 2 apologises again and exits.

   > **Teaching Point**: *These changes in role on the part of the teacher must be clearly signalled to the group.*

- Teacher re-enters out of role. Use narrative to describe the frustration of the group. Ask the group where they would like the birds' family to be. Listen to and accept ideas, selecting one. (A cave, a cliff, a tree, a mountain are likely suggestions.)

- Ask the group if they will now be the bird's family. Practice birdlike movements and sounds. Ask the group to find a place in the cave, on the cliff, in the tree, according to the suggestion that was selected.

- Bring the group together again (out of role) and ask them how the lost bird would find her own family. Listen to and accept ideas, selecting a few for enactment. Get the group to practice these ideas and send them back, as birds, to their cave, cliff, tree.

- The adult in role as the lost bird can now enact the search, listening for the sounds or other signs that have been suggested.

Teaching Point: *Tension can be developed if the T/F sets the scene by using narrative to suggest that at first the sounds or other signs were very faint. Perhaps the birds will make quiet bird sounds, perhaps just one or two birds fly out then return. The adult in role as the bird can then, gradually, enact the moment of finding her own family. The tension can be extended if the T/F, again using narrative, says that the bird discovered where its family were, but could not get to them. Out of role, the children can decide how that could occur and can enact the moment of reconciliation. The T/F will need to structure this moment so the adult in role as the bird is protected.*

- The bird is re-united with its family. It says it is very tired and asks the other birds to use birdsong to sing it to sleep.

- T/F uses narrative to say that as the song continued, all the bird fell asleep, happy that their lost one had returned.

- Bring the group (out of role) back into a gathered group. Use narrative (briefly) to complete the story. 'So the bird and its family were re-united, thanks to the help of the ornithologists and when the next winter came and the birds were preparing to fly off to X, they made quite sure that every one of them was there before they set off on their journey.'

PLAN SIX

This plan was devised for a two to three year old group. The group had been considering various aspects of colours. The teachers were interested in observing drama strategies that were appropriate for young children.

Only one teacher was available to take roles in this drama. This plan gives some suggestions as to what the teacher can do if there are no responses at all from the children.

Topic: Colours, particularly of plants and flowers

Role for children: Gardeners

Role for adult: Lady who has planted a garden plus other roles as suggested by the children

Focus/problem: The plants in a garden are changing colour in inappropriate ways.

What are the learning objectives?

To engage two to three year olds in the drama contexts of situation, role, symbol and space through improvisation, narrative and movement.

To draw upon children's knowledge of colours and colour combinations

Teaching/learning process

- Begin with children in a circle or gathered group. Explain that in drama we take roles and accept that we are in a variety of places. (See earlier plans.)

- Indicate that in today's drama, the children will be gardeners. Get agreement.

- T/F exits and re-enters in role as someone who needs the help of some expert gardeners. This character expresses relief that she has found the right people and asks what sorts of gardening they know about. Could they show her some of the things they do when they are being gardeners?

> **Teaching Point**: *If the children do not respond, the character can lead them into enactment by saying things like 'I suppose you'd need to be digging. Could you show me what you do when you are digging. Do you do it this way?' As digging is demonstrated, the children are likely to copy and the character can say 'Yes, that's how I usually dig, too. What about watering. Do you use a hose?' This is only likely to be necessary with very young children.*

- After a few gardening activities have been enacted, sit the group down again. The character says, 'Oh I am glad I found you. You do seem to know a lot about gardening.'

- The character presents the problem by explaining she has planted a garden but everything has grown the wrong colour.

  > **Teaching Point**: *Character should elaborate here by describing the plants and indicating what has happened to them. Red roses have turned orange, the green grass is blue, etc.*

- Listen to and accept ideas.

  > **Teaching Point**: *If no ideas at all are forthcoming (although this will be unlikely if there are at least some children in the group who are verbal) the character can shake her head and say something like, 'Yes, it is strange, isn't it. I don't understand it either.'*

- Character asks if the gardeners would come with her to see her garden for themselves.

- Character says her garden is a long way away and wonders how the gardeners will get there, Listen to suggestions and select one.

  > **Teaching Point**: *If no ideas are given the character may simply suggest they all go in a bus. 'If I get a bus to come round, I think we'd all fit in.'*

- Enact the journey (See Chapter Five).

- On arrival at the garden the character presents the problem again, showing the gardeners around, pointing out and describing the ways the colours have changed.

    > **Teaching Point**: *This provides opportunities for movement as the character enacts the movements as they are described. 'If you stretch up and look over here, you can see that the climbing roses are purple and they should be pink. If you just crawl through this archway, you can tell that the ferns are yellow and they should be green'.*

- Listen to and accept any comments that are made.

- Character says, 'It looks to me as if someone has come in here and changed all those colours, but I don't know who it is.' Listen to and accept ideas. If a specific person is suggested, the teacher takes that role, coached by the children.

- Using narrative, teacher (out of role) says that at night, when everyone was asleep, someone came into the garden.

- Gardeners all lie down and close their eyes.

- T/F says that now she is going to be the person who changed all the colours in the garden.

- In role as the character suggested, the teacher comes in and, using movement and dialogue, demonstrates how the colours were changed and then exits.

    > **Teaching Point**: *One group decided the colours were changed because someone called Jack came in at night at painted everything. In this case, this is what was re-enacted. If the children have made no suggestions at all, a scene can still be enacted. After the children have watched this scene, the T/F can say 'So you see what happened'*

- Teacher resumes role as the character with a garden and asks the gardeners how this person could be prevented from damaging the garden.

- Listen to and accept idea, choosing one or a combination of ideas to be enacted.

> **Teaching Point**: *The scene in which the person who damaged the garden is dealt with needs careful handling. The actions selected need to be enacted to the satisfaction of the children but in ways that protect the teacher. A possible strategy is to get the children to enact their ideas but without the perpetrator present. Then the children can sit down and watch the teacher in role as the person who damaged the garden re-enact the scene, using narrative, movement and dialogue, but without the children being engaged in the action. This formalisation of the scene can be effective, enjoyable and safe.*

- The character who has damaged the garden exits.

- The teacher again takes the role of the owner of the garden and shakes hands with each gardener, thanking them for their assistance.

- Finally, all sit in a circle or gathered group, as at the beginning of the drama. The teacher (now out of role) uses narrative to bring the story to an end.

PLAN SEVEN

This plan uses a well known children's book, Where The Wild Things Are *by Maurice Sendak, as its starting point. The drama was initially developed by an early childhood teacher, Patricia Connolly, for use with a pre-school group and is used here with her permission. There are many possibilities for adaptation. Any character can be found in an unexpected or unsuitable situation and need assistance in returning to where it belongs.*

Topic: Developed from *Where The Wild Things Are* by Maurice Sendak.

Roles for Children: Coastguards. (alternatively the children could be to cast as people who live near Max and his mother).

Role/s for Adult/s: Max's mother or father/ Wild Things

Focus/Problem: Max's mother (or father) finds a Wild Thing asleep in Max'a boat.

What are the learning objectives?

To engage the children in the dramatic contexts of role, situation, symbol and mood through the forms of improvisation, movement and oral scripting.

To involve children in solving problems and in making decisions which will forward the course of the drama

Teaching/learning process

- Explain the ways in which drama allows for role taking and the acceptance of fictional situations.

- Make clear to the children that another adult will be taking a role in the drama and they will find out later just who he/she will be. The first time they meet the character, this person will be asleep in the bottom of a small boat.

- Ask the group what could be used to signify a boat. Get agreement and ask the adult to lie down in that boat as if asleep.

- Explain to the group that in the drama, they will be taking the role of coastguards, people who know a lot about the sea.

    Teaching Point: *It is also possible to tell the children they need to be people who know a lot about boats and about the sea and to ask their advice about appropriate roles. Listen to and accept ideas, selecting one that is suitable.*

- T/F exits, explaining that when he/she r-enters, the drama will begin.

- Character re-enters in search of coastguards (or the role that has been decided upon). Expresses relief that they are those people. Explains that Max has a small boat and likes to sail off to a nearby island. He came home, just as he usually does, but when the character (Max's mother or father) went down to check on the boat, there was a Wild Thing, fast asleep in the bottom of the boat. What is to be done?

- Listen to, accept and extend ideas.

    Teaching Point: *If children have not suggested it, mother/father asks if they would come and look for themselves. All move across to the boat. Character asks again what should be done.*

- If necessary, lead to towards waking the Wild Thing although it is better if the children suggest this themselves. They are likely to do so if given time. Children suggest how this is done and a few strategies are tried before one is successful. The Wild Thing should wake slowly, look perturbed at the watching crowd and begin to cry softly.

- Group discuss what the problem could be. They can question the Wild Thing and eventually work out that it did not mean to fall asleep in the boat and wants to get back before the Wild Rumpus.

    Teaching Point: *It is best if the children can be led to this conclusion rather than have the Wild Thing tell them the problem immediately.*

- Mother/father wonders what should be done. When the children suggest taking or sending the Wild Thing back, express concern as to how this could be done. Wild Thing expresses fear about going back by itself and mother/father worries that Max's boat is not big enough for them all.

- Listen to and suggest ideas. Select an appropriate course of action, from the ideas put forward by the children, and enact it.

    Teaching Point: *If the children suggest a bigger boat, the procuring of this boat needs to be considered and difficulties discussed, After all, a large boat cannot (and should not) appear as if by magic.*

- When the group arrive on the island, teacher can indicate he/she will change roll, exiting and returning as another Wild Thing who blames the group for taking the first Wild Thing away.

    Teaching Point: *This role should not be too scary. This Wild Thing should be cross but not furious.*

- If the children do not respond, Max's mother/father can react to this undeserved attack. 'Why does it think it is our fault?' could be a useful question.

- Suggest the group explain what happened.

- Now this Wild Thing turns to the Wild Thing who was in the boat and scolds it for being so careless, saying it cannot take part in the Wild Rumpus.

- Wild Thing crumples, crying softly and says it really wanted to dance at the Wild Rumpus.

- Max's mother/father wonders what could be done to persuade the cross Wild Thing let the other one join the Wild Rumpus. Listen to and accept ideas

    Teaching Point: *A conversation between the group and the Wild Things could be orally scripted and then enacted (See Chapter Five) and can lead to the second Wild Thing relenting.*

- The Wild Thing from the boat asks if its rescuers could come as well and this is agreed on.

- The wild rumpus is enacted.

> **Teaching Point**: *Music can be used. This final scene can be a general free flowing dance or it can be formalised. If the latter, the second Wild Thing can introduce the Wild Rumpus as a celebratory ritual that must follow certain rules. As the ritual proceeds the group should be invited to lead by suggesting how the performance should progress.*

- Something signals the end of the Wild Rumpus. (a loud sound, a bell or a gong or it can be visual – eg one of the Wild Things runs round the group with a banner or flag). Wild Thing says they must all leave the island. Narrative can cover the return journey or it can be enacted.

- The group sits down and the teacher, out of role, uses narrative to conclude the story.

CHAPTER NINE

EPILOGUE

SOME FINAL THOUGHTS

The skills and strategies discussed in this book as those which will contribute to effective drama teaching, are also skills, which, once acquired, will remain with teachers and extend to all their work with children. After teachers have used questions that ask children for their opinions, their 'interpretation of ideas' (Wagner, 1976 p.65) they will be less interested in asking narrowly focussed questions and never again will they use questions which demand the children guess what the teacher is thinking. They will not be afraid to allow the children *time to consider* and they will not find it necessary to answer their own questions. When teachers ask questions as if they want to know the answers and are willing to wait while the children think about the possible ramifications of the issues raised, they free children to share their ideas and their understanding of the world, providing valuable insights into their interpretations of reality.

The educational values and assumptions that inspire process drama are derived from the right children have to an education that acknowledges their need to own their own learning, that empowers them and that allows and encourages them to understand the world in which they live (Norman, 1999 p.9). Drama is a significant medium through which teachers can explore children's conceptual, experiential and emotional worlds (Warren, 2000 p.128). But drama is more than an educational tool; it is an art form in its own right (Crooks, 1998 p.27) and this book has constantly reflected the ways in which process drama and theatre are intertwined. As O'Neill (1994 p.152) suggests, theatre and process drama share structure, form and purpose. Both 'generate significant meanings and raise significant questions.'

This book has lead its readers through ways of planning and implementing process drama experiences with young children of all ages and abilities. Examples have been provided to illumine the practical suggestions given. The theories that underlie practice have been considered. Some sample plans have been included along with suggestions for their implementation.

The success of drama, however, must lie in its performance. As teachers and children engage in making, performing and appreciating drama, they will discover more about the excitement and power of the art form and will share the 'pleasure and zeal' that O'Toole (1998 p.15) believes is common to all teachers of drama. They will recognise its affiliation with developmentally appropriate practice and will value its potential to make powerful and authentic contributions to children's learning. They will experience the excitement of a successful drama experience and will come out of those lessons with a feeling of exhilaration. They, like drama teachers all over the world, will be 'hooked on drama'.

BIBLIOGRAPHY

Arthur, L., Beecher, B., Docket, S., Farmer, S. & Richards, E. (1993). *Programming and Planning in Early Childhood Settings*. Sydney: Harcourt Brace.

Aston, L. (1996). Interview with the author.

Barnes, H. (1998). Identifying educational strategies for use with deaf pupils. *Drama; J. of National Drama*. 5 (3). 20-25.

Belcher, J. (1996). Interview with the author.

Bolton, G. (1984). Teacher in role and teacher power. Unpublished paper cited in C. O'Neill. *Drama Worlds; A Framework for Process Drama*. Portsmouth, N.H.: Heinemann.

Bolton, G. (1992). *New Perspectives on Classroom Drama*. London: Simon and Schuster.

Bolton, G. (1997, July). A conceptual framework for classroom acting. Keynote address given at *Second International Drama in Education Research* Institute. University of Victoria, Canada.

Booth, D. (1987). *Drama Words*. Toronto, Canada: Language Study Centre, Drama.

Booth, D. (1993, September).Closing address at Conference on *The Relationship between Drama and Learning: An International Research Conference. Institue of Education, University of London*. England.

Booth, D. (1997, July). Discussions held during *Second International Drama in Education Research Institute*. University of Victoria, Canada.

Bruner, J. (1988). Vygotsky: A historical and conceptual perspective. In N. Mercer (Ed.)*Language and Literacy from an Educational perspective*. *Vol.1*. 86-98. Milton Keynes: Open University Press.

Bruner, J. (1990). *Acts of Meaning*. Cambridge, Mass.: Harvard University Press.

Carroll, J. (1988). Terra Incognita: mapping drama talk. *National Association for Drama in Education J. (Aust.)*.12 (2) 13-20.

Carroll, J. (1993, July). Drama as radical pedagogy. Paper presented at *Conference to Celebrate the Work and Influence of Dorothy Heathcote*. Lancaster, England.

Clyde, M. & Fleet, A. (1993). *What's in a Day? Working in early Childhood*. Katoomba, Australia: Social Science Press.

Cohen, R. (1988). *Theatre: Brief version*. (2nd edn.). California: Mayfield.

Crooks, J. (1998). Working in a school-university partnership: a mentor's perspective *Drama: J. of National Drama.* 6(1). 27-31.

Cross, T. (1997). Developmentally appropriate practice: new ways to go. In S. Wyver, T. Cross & G. Lewis (Eds.). *Selected papers from Three Child Development Conferences.* Sydney: Centre for Child Development, Macquarie University.

Cupit, G. (1989). Socialising the superheroes. *Resource Booklet No.5.* Canberra: Australian Early Childhood Association.

Dau, E. (1991). Let's pretend: sociodramatic play in early childhood. In S. Wright (Ed.), *The Arts in Early Childhood.* Sydney: Prentice Hall.

Davies, G. (1983). *Practical Primary Drama.* London: Heinemann.

Davis, S. (1998). *Gender Equity Policy and Guidelines.* National Association for drama in Education (Aust.).

Dawkins, M. (1991). Hey dude's, what's the rap? A pleas for leniency towards superhero play. *Australian J. Early Childhood.* 12 (2). 3-8.

Derman-Sparkes, L. (1991, September). An anti-bias curriculum: tools for empowering children. Paper given at *The Nineteenth National Conference of the Australian Early Childhood Association.* Adelaide: Australia.

Dunn, L. (1995). A voice from the ground. IDEA'95 Australian teacher's keynote address. *National Association for Drama in Education J. (Aust).* 19 (2), 3-13.

Dunn, J. (1996). Spontaneous Dramatic Play and the 'Super-dramatist: who's structuring the elements of dramatic form. *National Association for Drama in Education J. (Aust).* 20 (2), 19-28.

Esslin, M. (1987). *The Field of Drama.* London: Methuen.

Fitzgibbon, E. (1997). Crossing the boundaries: drama as subject and method. *Drama Matters. J. of Ohio Drama Education Exchange.* 2 (1), 5-18.

Fleming, K. (1994). *Starting Drama Teaching.* London: David Fulton.

Forehan, B. (1991). Drama with Visually impaired children. *National Association* for Drama in Education J. (Aust). 15 (2). 11-15.

Gates, N. (1996). Interview with the author.

Gifford, M. (1997, June). What is a good play? Paper given *at Annual Seminar of* the *Speech and Drama Association of New South Wales.* Sydney: Australia.

Gronlund, G. (1992). Coping with Ninja Turtle play in my kindergarten. *Young Children.* 48 (1). 21-25.

Hasemans, B. & O'Toole, J. (1986). *Dramawise: An Introduction to the Elements of Drama*. Melbourne: Heinemann Educational.

Heathcote, D. (1967). Improvisation. In L. Johnson & C. O'Neill (Eds.). (1984). *Dorothy Heathcote: Collected Writings on Education and Drama*. London: Hutchinson.

Heathcote, D. (1978). Drama and the mentally handicapped. In L. Johnson & C. O'Neill (Eds.). *Dorothy Heathcote: Collected Writings on Education and Drama*. London: Hutchinson.

Heathcote, D. (1984). Drama as context for talking and writing. In L. Johnson & C. O'Neill (Eds.). *Dorothy Heathcote: Collected Writings on Education and Drama*. London: Hutchinson.

Heathcote, D. (1985). Personal tutorials with Dorothy Heathcote. Newcastle-upon-Tyne, UK. (Based on discussions between the author and Heathcote.) Unpublished.

Heathcote, D. with Bell, E., Bowmaker, H., Chilley, M., Gibbon, Oakes, S., Pivars, M. & Vause, M. (1988). in T. Roberts (Ed.). *Drama in Encouraging Expression: The Arts in the Primary Curriculum*. London: Cassell.

Heathcote, D. & Bolton, G. (1994). *Drama for Learning; Dorothy Heathcote's Mantle of the Expert Approach to Education*. Portsmouth, N.H.: Heinemann.

Heathcote, D. & Pennington, E. (1989). Dramatic symbol and mantle of the expert. *National Association for Drama in Education J. (Aust.)*. 14 (1) 2-9

Howe, J. (1999). *Early Childhood, Family and Society in Australia. A Reassessment*. Katoomba, Australia: Social Science Press.

Human Rights and Equal Opportunities Commission. (1997). *Bringing Then Home: the Report of the National Inquiry into the Separation of Aboriginal and Torres Strait Islander Childhood From Their Families*. Canberra: Australian Government.

Knowles, B. (1999). Personal communication.

Johnson, J., Christie, J. & Yawkey, T. (1987). *Play and Early Childhood Development*. Illinois: Scott Forseman.

Lanning, B. (1989). Theatre for the visually handicapped. *London Drama Magazine*. November. 10-11.

McNaughton, M.J. (1998). Inquiry learning through drama with young children. *Drama: J. of National Drama*. 6 (1). 10-16.

Makin, L., Campbell, J. & Jones-Diaz, C. (1995). *One Childhood, Many Languages*. Sydney: Harper Educational.

Morgan, N. & Saxton, J. (1987). *Teaching Drama; A Mind if Many Wonders*. London: Hutchinson.

Morgan, N. & Saxton, J. (1991a). Well, if I called the wrong number, why did you answer the 'phone? *Drama Contact*. 15. Autumn. 13-15.

Morgan, N. & Saxton, J. (1991). *Teaching Questioning, Learning*. London: Routledge.

Morgan, N. (1997, October). Integrating the arts: drama, art, P.T. & Music. Workshop given at *Dramaxix; Positioning Drama: NADIE Conference*. Sydney: Australia.

Neelands, J. (1984). *Making Sense of Drama*. London: Heinemann.

Neelands, J. & Goode, T. (1995). Playing in the margins of meaning: the ritual aesthetic in community performance. *National Association for Drama in Education J. (Aust.)*. 10 (1). 39-56.

New South Wales Board of Studies (1998). *Creative Arts; K-6 Draft Syllabus and Support Documents*. Sydney: NSW Board of Studies.

Nixon, D. & Aldwinkle, M. (1997). *Exploring Child Development from Three to Six Years*. Katoomba, Aust.: Social Science Press.

Norman, J. (1999). Brain right drama. *Drama: J. of National Drama*. 6 (2). 8-13.

O'Neill, C. (1990). Course for teachers held at London Drama, London. (Unpublished).

O'Neill, C. (1994). Here comes everybody: aspects of role in process drama. *National Association for Drama in Education J. (Aust), International Research Edition*. 18 (2), 37-44.

O'Neill, C. (1995). *Drama Worlds: A Framework for Process Drama*. Portsmouth, N.H. Heinemann.

O'Toole, J. (1992). *The Process of Drama: Negotiating Art and Meaning*. London: Routledge.

O'Toole, J. (1998). Playing on the beach: consensus among drama teachers – some patterns in the sand. *National Association for Drama in Education J. (Aust.)*. 22 (2) 5-20.

Parsons, B., Schaffner, M., Little, G. & Felton, H. (1984). *Drama Language and Learning*. National Association for Drama in Education Papers. No 1. Hobart: National Association for Drama in Education.

Parsons, B. (1991). Story-making and drama for children 5-8 years. In S.Wright (Ed.) *The Arts in Early Childhood*. Sydney: Prentice Hall.

Pena, S. French, J. & Holmes, R. (1987). A look at superheroes: some issues and guidelines. *Day Care and Early Education*. 15 (1). 10-14.

Perlmutter, J. & Pellegrini, A. (1989). Parental distancing strategies and children's fantasy play. In M. Bloch and A. Pellegrini (Eds.). *The Ecological Context of Children's Play*. New Jersey: Ablex. 155-162.

Peters, M. (1994). *Drama For All: Developing Drama in the Curriculum with Pupils with Special Educational Needs*. London: David Fulton.

Phillips, A. (1993). *The Trouble With Boys: Parenting the Men of the Future*. London: Pandora.

Rabinov, P. (Ed.). (1984). *The Foucalt Reader: an Introduction to Foucalt's Thought*. London: Penguin.

Rowe, M. (1996). Wait time: slowing down may be a way of speeding up. *J. of teacher Education*. Jan/Feb. 43-50.

Schaffner, M. (1984). Language development through drama. In B. Parsons, M. Schaffner, G. Little & H. Felton (1984) National Association for Drama in Education Papers. No 1. Hobart: National Association for Drama in Education.

Sendak, M. (1975). *Where the Wild Things Are*. London: Bodley Head.

Simons, J. (1991). Concept development and drama: scaffolding the learning. In J, Hughes (Ed.). *Drama in Education: The State of the Art*. Sydney: Educational Drama Association of New South Wales.

Stewart, C. & Cash, W. (1988). *Interviewing: Principles and Practice*. (5th Edn.) Iowa: Wm.C. Brown.

Tandy. M. (1993). Beyond e.g.: primary teachers as teachers of drama. *Drama: One Forum, Many Voices: J. of National Drama*. 1 (3) 2-6.

Tough, J. (1977). *The Development of Meaning*. London: Unwin.

Turnbull, J. (1988). Music. in T. Roberts (Ed.) *Special Needs in Ordinary Schools: Encouraging Expression. Arts in the Primary Curriculum*. London: Cassell.

Vygotsky, L. (1978). The development of higher psychological processes. In *Mind and Society*. Cambridge, Mass.: Harvard University Press.

Wagner, B-J. (1976). *Dorothy Heathcote: Drama As a Learning Medium*. Washington: National Education Association.

Warren, K. (1994, July). An examination of pre-school children's ideas and impressions of the superheroes: some implications for gender education. In *Voicing Our Agendas: Gender and Teacher Education Conference Papers.* Ubud: Bali.

Warren, K. (1995). Everyone succeeds in drama. *Drama Contact.* 19. Autumn. 34-40.

Warren, K. (1997). Using drama with children with special needs. In S. Wyver, T. Cross & G. Lewis (Eds.). *Selected Papers From Three Child Development Conferences.* Sydney: Centre for Child Development, Macquarie University.

Warren, K. (1998). *Early Childhood Teachers' Understanding and Practice of Drama.* Unpublished Doctoral Dissertation. Sydney: Macquarie University.

Warren, K. (2000). Thinking for the new millenium: the contribution of process drama. In W. Schiller (Ed.). *Thinking Through the Arts.* Sydney: Fine Arts Press. (To be published, 2000.)

Watts, D. (1986). The plight of the taken male. *Times Educational Supplement.* 14th November. P.22.

Winston, J. (1996). Drama and emergent writing: a case study. *Australian Drama Education Magazine.* 2. 22-27.

Winston, J. (1998). 'Should we follow Jack?' A case study of reflective practitioner research into drama and moral education. *National Association for Drama in Education j. (Aust).* 22 (1). 19-25.

Wood, D. (1986). Aspects of teaching and learning. In M.Richards & P. Light (Eds.). *Children of Social Worlds.* Cambridge, Mass.: Harvard University Press.